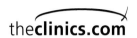

HEART FAILURE CLINICS

The Role of Surgery, Part I

GUEST EDITORS
Stephen Westaby, MS, PhD
Mario C. Deng, MD

CONSULTING EDITORS
Jagat Narula, MD, PhD
James B. Young, MD

April 2007 • Volume 3 • Number 2

SAUNDERS

An Imprint of Elsevier, Inc.
PHILADELPHIA   LONDON   TORONTO   MONTREAL   SYDNEY   TOKYO

W.B. SAUNDERS COMPANY

A Division of Elsevier Inc.

1600 John F. Kennedy Boulevard. • Suite 1800 • Philadelphia, Pennsylvania 19103-2899

http://www.theclinics.com

HEART FAILURE CLINICS
April 2007
Editor: Barbara Cohen-Kligerman

Volume 3, Number 2
ISSN 1551-7136
ISBN-13: 978-1-4160-4321-8
ISBN-10: 1-4160-4321-7

Reprints: For copies of 100 or more, or articles in this publication, please contact the Commercial Reprints Department, Elsevier Inc., 360 Park Avenue South, New York, New York 10010-1710. Tel.: (+1) 212-633-3813; Fax: (+1) 212-462-1935; e-mail: reprints@elsevier.com.

The ideas and opinions expressed in *Heart Failure Clinics* do not necessarily reflect those of the Publisher. The Publisher does not assume any responsibility for any injury and/or damage to persons or property arising out of or related to any use of the material contained in this periodical. The reader is advised to check the appropriate medical literature and the product information currently provided by the manufacturer of each drug to be administered to verify the dosage, the method and duration of administration, or contraindications. It is the responsibility of the treating physician or other health care professional, relying on independent experience and knowledge of the patient, to determine drug dosages and the best treatment for the patient. Mention of any product in this issue should not be construed as endorsement by the contributors, editors, or the Publisher of the product or manufacturers' claims.

Heart Failure Clinics (ISSN 1551-7136) is published quarterly by Elsevier Inc., 360 Park Avenue South, New York, NY 10010-1710. Months of publication are January, April, July, and October. Business and editorial offices: 1600 John F. Kennedy Boulevard, Suite 1800, Phliadelphia, PA 19103-2899. Customer service office: 6277 Sea Harbor Drive, Orlando, FL 32887-4800. Periodicals postage paid at New York, NY and additional mailing offices. Subscription prices are USD 157 per year for US individuals, USD 260 per year for US institutions, USD 54 per year for US students and residents, USD 189 per year for Canadian individuals, USD 292 per year for Canadian institutions, USD 189 per year for international individuals, USD 292 per year for international institutions and USD 65 per year for foreign students/residents. To receive student and resident rate, orders must be accompanied by name of affiliated institution, date of term, and the *signature* of program/residency coordinator on institution letterhead. Orders will be billed at individual rate until proof of status is received. Foreign air speed delivery is included in all *Clinics* subscription prices. All prices are subject to change without notice. POSTMASTER: Send address changes to *Heart Failure Clinics*, Elsevier Periodicals Customer Service, 6277 Sea Harbor Drive, Orlando, FL 32887-4800. **Customer Service: 1-800-654-2452 (US). From outside of the US, call (+1) 407-345-4000.**

Heart Failure Clinics is covered in *Index Medicus*.

Printed in the United States of America.

Cover artwork courtesy of Umberto M. Jezek.

CONSULTING EDITORS

JAGAT NARULA, MD, PhD, Professor, Medicine; Chief, Division of Cardiology; and Associate Dean, University of California Irvine School of Medicine, Irvine, California

JAMES B. YOUNG, MD, Chairman and Professor, Department of Medicine, Lerner College of Medicine; and George and Linda Kaufman Chair, Cleveland Clinic Foundation, Case Western Reserve University, Cleveland, Ohio

GUEST EDITORS

STEPHEN WESTABY, MS, PhD, FRCS, Professor, Oxford Heart Centre, John Radcliffe Hospital, Headington, Oxford, United Kingdom

MARIO C. DENG, MD, FACC, FESC, Director of Cardiac Transplantation Research, Columbia University, Department of Medicine, Division of Cardiology, New York, New York

CONTRIBUTORS

L. BALACUMARASWAMI, MBBS, FRCS (C-Th), Oxford Heart Centre, John Radcliffe Hospital, Headington, Oxford, United Kingdom

CHRISTINA CHO, BA, Research Assistant, Department of Medicine, Division of Cardiology, Center for Interventional Vascular Therapies, College of Physicians and Surgeons, Columbia University, Columbia University Medical Center, New York, New York

GEORGE M. COMAS, MD, Cardiothoracic Research Fellow, Division of Cardiothoracic Surgery, College of Physicians and Surgeons, Columbia University, New York, New York

MARISA DI DONATO, MD, Department of Critical Care Medicine, University of Florence, Firenze, Italy

BARRY C. ESRIG, MD, Attending in Surgery, Division of Cardiothoracic Surgery, College of Physicians and Surgeons, Columbia University, New York, New York

O.H. FRAZIER, MD, Director of the Center for Cardiac Support, Texas Heart Institute at St. Luke's Episcopal Hospital; and Professor of Surgery, Baylor College of Medicine, Houston, Texas

AJAY J. KIRTANE, MD, SM, Assistant Professor of Clinical Medicine, Center for Interventional Vascular Therapy, Division of Cardiology, Columbia University Medical Center; and Director of Clinical Biometrics, Data Coordinating and Analysis Center, Cardiovascular Research Foundation, New York, New York

TIMOTHY P. MARTENS, MD, Associate Research Scientist, Division of Cardiothoracic Surgery, Department of Surgery; and Department of Biomedical Engineering, College of Physicians and Surgeons, Columbia University, New York, New York

LORENZO MENICANTI, MD, Department of Cardiac Surgery, San Donato Hospital, San Donato Milanese, Milano, Italy

JEFFREY W. MOSES, MD, Professor of Medicine; Director, Center for Interventional Vascular Therapy; and Director, Cardiac Catheterization Laboratories, Columbia University Medical Center, New York, New York

MEHMET C. OZ, MD, Professor of Surgery, Division of Cardiothoracic Surgery, College of Physicians and Surgeons, Columbia University, New York, New York

SORIN V. PUSCA, MD, Clinical Instructor, Cardiothoracic Surgery, Emory Heart Center, Division of Cardiothoracic Surgery, Emory University School of Medicine, Emory Crawford Long Hospital, Atlanta, Georgia

JOHN D. PUSKAS, MD, Associate Chief of Cardiothoracic Surgery and Chief of Cardiac Surgery, Emory Heart Center, Division of Cardiothoracic Surgery, Emory University School of Medicine, Emory Crawford Long Hospital, Atlanta, Georgia

HIND RAHMOUNI, MD, Division of Cardiology, University of Pennsylvania Medical Center, Philadelphia, Pennsylvania

R. SAYEED, PhD, FRCS, Oxford Heart Centre, John Radcliffe Hospital, Headington, Oxford, United Kingdom

WARREN SHERMAN, MD, FACC, FSCAI, Director, Cardiac Cell-Based Endovascular Therapies, Department of Medicine, Division of Cardiology, Center for Interventional Vascular Therapies, College of Physicians and Surgeons, Columbia University, Columbia University Medical Center, New York, New York

SARA J. SHUMWAY, MD, Professor, Cardiovascular and Thoracic Surgery, Department of Surgery, University of Minnesota, Minneapolis, Minnesota

MARTIN ST. JOHN SUTTON, MD, FRCP, Division of Cardiology, University of Pennsylvania Medical Center, Philadelphia, Pennsylvania

STEPHEN WESTABY, MS, PhD, FRCS, Professor, Oxford Heart Centre, John Radcliffe Hospital, Headington, Oxford, United Kingdom

CONTENTS

FORTHCOMING ISSUES

RECENT ISSUES

THE CLINICS ARE NOW AVAILABLE ONLINE!

Access your subscription at:
http://www.theclinics.com

ELSEVIER
SAUNDERS

Heart Failure Clin 3 (2007) ix–x

HEART
FAILURE
CLINICS

Editorial

Surgical Intervention in Heart Failure: Observing Obedience to the Nature

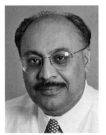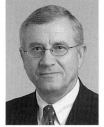

Jagat Narula, MD, PhD   James B. Young, MD
Consulting Editors

Since there is a distinct relationship between left ventricular (LV) volume and outcomes, ventricular reduction or "remodeling" surgery has been proposed as a corrective intervention in heart failure. These approaches decrease ventricular chamber dilation and may eliminate dyskinesia. Of various surgical approaches, the "Batista" and "Dor" procedures have raised both excitement and controversy. Rather than debating the merits (and limitations) of such procedures, it is important to address whether the morphoanatomy of LV is even amenable to ventricular volume reduction by surgical remodeling.

J. Bell Pettigrew, in 1864, very eloquently pointed out that the left ventricular myocardium is exceedingly simple in principle, but wonderfully complicated in detail. The arrangement of the LV myocardial fibers has been described as descending and ascending bands, laminated layers, or right- and left-handed helical arrangements that correspond to the subendocardial and subepicardial myocardium [1]. The fibers in the endocardial and epicardial blankets are counterdirectional, and shortening of these mantles of muscle fibers results in a wringing movement of the LV. The peculiar morphoanatomy of the LV displays both inflow and outflow lying side by side at the base of the heart, and a unique sequence of electrical activation and myocardial contraction becomes necessary to direct the flow pattern discretely and smoothly through the ventricle during systole and diastole.

Recent studies of LV activation and contraction have demonstrated that the apical subendocardium is the first to be activated followed by basal subendocardium, and then apical and basal epicardium [2]. Consequently, contraction from the apical to basal subendocardium in isovolumic contraction phase sets the direction of blood flow toward outflow tract. This isovolumic contraction sequence also results in a minor clockwise twist of the apex. Subsequent contraction of the apical epicardium gradually extends to the basal epicardium and forces the vertical epicardial mantle of myocardium into a more horizontal orientation, which reduces longitudinal axial dimensions, pulls the base toward the apex, and results in systolic ejection. The apex twists substantially in counterclockwise direction during the ejection phase. Relaxation then begins at the apical endocardium electromechanically before the base. The longer contraction of the basal endocardium ensures evacuation of the subvalvular regions, while the relaxing apical segment allows blood flow toward the apex, preparing it for receiving diastolic filling. Subsequent relaxation of the basal epicardium allows unopposed contraction of apical epicardium that untwists the apex (clockwise rotation) and restores the fiber geometry to elongate the LV longitudinal axis. The continued and isolated epicardial contraction coincides with isovolumic relaxation period and extends to the early rapid filling phase. Elongation of the ventricular longitudinal dimension sets up suction and indicates that at least early diastole is an active process; slow filling occurs passively.

Recent elegant descriptions and clarification of the sequential myocardial electromechanical activation has significant surgical implications. Surgical LV volume reduction and remodeling in patients who have ischemic and non-ischemic dilated cardiomyopathy, therefore, deserve careful consideration. Though surgical approaches to restoring a more normal contractile geometry in the LV are intuitively attractive, it is likely that long-term success will be dependent upon preserving the unique electromechanical activation and relaxation pattern. The marvelous and seemingly paradoxic simplicity of the myofiber arrangement complexity demands that surgeons observe obedience to the nature of the ventricle. Professor Westaby and Dr. Deng bring to us the rather extraordinary advances in surgical interventions for management of complicated heart failure, and coax readers not to give up!

Jagat Narula, MD, PhD
University of California, Irvine, CA, USA

E-mail address: narula@uci.edu

James B. Young, MD
Cleveland Clinic Foundation, Cleveland, OH, USA

E-mail address: youngj@ccf.org

References

[1] Narula J, Vannan MA, DeMaria AN. Of that Waltz in my heart. J Am Coll Cardiol 2007;49(8):917–20.
[2] Sengupta PP, Khandheria BK, Korinek J, et al. Left ventricular isovolumic flow sequence during sinus and paced rhythms: new insights from use of high-resolution Doppler and ultrasonic digital particle imaging velocimetry. J Am Coll Cardiol 2007;49(8): 899–908.

HEART
FAILURE
CLINICS

Heart Failure Clin 3 (2007) xi–xiii

Preface

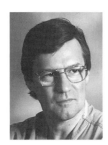
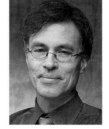

Stephen Westaby, MS, PhD, FRCS   Mario C. Deng, MD, FACC, FESC
Guest Editors

Worldwide, the heart failure syndrome has been increasing over the past decades, mainly because of the improved survival in acute heart attack situations in industrialized societies, as well as the epidemiologic transition in major parts of the world. The prevalence of heart failures is estimated to be around 1%–3% of the population. The advanced heart failure fraction of this group is estimated at 10%. In the United States of America and Europe alone, out of each population of greater than 300 million inhabitants, 3 to 5 million people who have heart failure and 300,000 to 500,000 people who have advanced heart failure have to face a situation with reduced survival probability that is worse than the average prognosis of cancer, as well as impaired quality of life and a functional status.

Over the last three decades, based on an increasingly sophisticated understanding of the pathophysiology of the heart failure syndrome, therapeutic interventions have been tested in randomized clinical trials and implemented into clinical practice. Foremost, these have included the concept of neurohormonal blockade, which inhibits the chronic activation of the adrenergic nervous system by way of beta blockade, as well as inhibits the chronic activation of the renin-

angiotensin-aldosterone system by angiotensin converting enzyme inhibitors, aldosterone receptor blockers, and aldosterone antagonists. Furthermore, interventional concepts, including defibrillator therapy and resynchronization pacemaker therapy, have been, after having shown survival and quality of life benefit, implemented in clinical practice.

With respect to surgical treatment options in advanced heart failure, the situation in terms of evidence-based medicine has been less clear. For example, although heart transplantation—based on the initial spectacular success by Norman Shumway and colleagues at Stanford University—has been implemented in 300 centers around the world, it was never tested in a randomized clinical trial. More recently, the role of mechanical circulatory support therapy has been shown to yield a survival and quality of life benefit in advanced heart failure patients who are ineligible for heart transplantation. However, all other surgical options, including coronary artery bypass surgery, valvular surgery, and left ventricular volume reduction surgery, are based on observational series. In this situation, we would like to contribute, with this issue, an update of the status of surgical therapy in heart failure in order to reflect the best current clinical practice patterns and clinical research directions. This issue comprises of a variety of articles that are provided by recognized authorities in their respective fields. Because of its overall volume, the issue is divided into Part I and Part II.

In the opening section, in the first article, Sara Shumway reflects on the lifetime achievement of her father, Norman Shumway, who spearheaded the era of cardiac transplantation in the 1950s and 1960s, and has been a role model in terms of clinical practice, translated from basic and clinical research. In the second article, Howard Frazier pays tribute to Michael DeBakey a pioneer in cardiac surgery who, while alive at the age of almost 100 years, has been considered a living icon for everyone involved in the field of cardiac surgery by pioneering cardiac surgical techniques and technology, and by developing heart mechanical support, heart biological replacement, and the classification of aortic dissecting aneurysms. With respect to the diagnostic imaging approach to the heart failure patient in preparation of cardiac surgery, the article by Martin St. John Sutton provides an expert evaluation of imaging techniques that allow for definition of interventional strategies and risk evaluation. In his articles, Stephen Westaby provides a provocative insight into the question of whether today's cardiac surgery is a therapy for all heart failure patients, and outlines strategies to maximize the benefit of high-risk cardiac surgery in heart failure patients.

In the second section on anti-ischemic surgical treatment options in heart failure, George Comas, Barry Esrig, and Mehmet C. Oz provide an insight into best practice patterns in patients who have acute coronary syndromes and life-threatening cardiogenic shock situations by surgical revascularization options. In the articles by Sorin V. Pusca and John D. Puscas, and by Ajay J. Kirtane and Jeffrey W. Moses, the debate on the topic of whether the cardiology interventional approaches with stent implantation or the cardiac surgical approach with coronary artery bypass grafting should be preferred is discussed. In their article, Lorenzo Menicanti and Marisa Di Donato outline the research scenario associated with the Surgical Treatment for Ischemic Heart Failure trial that is attempting to answer the question of whether a revascularization approach with or without left ventricular volume restoration in heart failure patients is superior to current best management practice. Concluding this section is the article by William Sherman and colleagues, which outlines rationales that are underway in order to improve

anti-ischemic treatment by stem cell transplantation at the time of surgical or cardiology interventional maneuvers.

In the third section of the issue, on antiarrhythmic and anti-pump failure interventions, Reynolds Delgado III and Howard Frazier advocate the left ventricular assist device approach for complete anti-arrhythmic treatment, while in their article, John Cleland, Abdellah Tageldien, Olga Khaleva, Neil Hobson, and Andrew L Clark argue for resynchronization therapy as a staged approach that has to precede more aggressive interventions. With respect to surgical treatment of hypertrophic cardiomyopathy, Anna Woo and Harry Rakowski summarize the experience utilizing myomectomy. In the final article of this section, Martinus Spoor[1] and Steven Bolling explain the rationales and analyze outcomes in patients who have advanced heart failure and are undergoing valve repair and replacement.

In the fourth section of the issue, in patients who have very advanced heart failure, beyond organ-saving anti-ischemic, anti–pump-failure, and anti-arrhythmic approaches, more complete heart replacement options are being discussed. Johannes Müeller argues in favor of a weaning attempt for recovery in every patient who has undergone mechanical circulatory support implantation, while Philip A. Poole-Wilson makes a point that the low rate of recovery does not justify this weaning protocol in every situation. For patients who are potential candidates for heart transplantation, Martin Cadeiras, Manuel von Bayern, and Mario C. Deng critically review the potential benefit of heart transplantation in the context of contemporary alternatives in contrast to the situation 30 years ago when heart transplantation was developed, as well as the challenges to improve long-term mechanical circulatory support outcomes by improving the technology associated with pump development. The final article, by Stephen Westaby, argues the pros and cons of expansion of destination mechanical circulatory support centers beyond the current transplant centers.

We hope—based on this comprehensive review of the current expertise in surgical therapies for advanced heart failure in the framework of the specific decision-making algorithm that we as a team are facing with our patients every day—that

---

[1] Martin Spoor, MD, died tragically in a plane crash on June 5, 2007 while retrieving a donor organ for heart transplantation.

this issue contributes to improvement in the field. We welcome your critical feedback.

Stephen Westaby, MS, PhD, FRCS
Oxford Heart Centre
John Radcliffe Hospital
Headley Way
Headington, Oxford OX3 9DU, UK

E-mail address: Stephen.westaby@orh.nhs.uk

Mario C. Deng, MD, FACC, FESC
Cardiac Transplantation Research
Department of Medicine
Division of Cardiology
Columbia University
622 West 168th Street
PH12 STEM, Room 134
New York, NY 10032, USA

E-mail address: md785@columbia.edu

ELSEVIER
SAUNDERS

HEART
FAILURE
CLINICS

Heart Failure Clin 3 (2007) 111–115

A Tribute to Norman E. Shumway, MD, PhD (1923–2006)

Sara J. Shumway, MD

Department of Surgery, University of Minnesota, Minneapolis, MN, USA

My father was a raconteur who led a storied life. Norman Edward Shumway (Figs. 1 and 2), Jr was born on February 9, 1923, to Norman Edward Shumway and Laura Irene VanderVliet Shumway. He was the only child of his generation in both families. His parents ran the Home Dairy in his hometown of Jackson, Michigan. It was a combination diner and creamery. Norman Edward Shumway, Sr also worked occasionally as an accountant. Bud, as he was known, was kicked out of a public pool at age 10 because he was not wearing a bathing suit that covered his chest. In later life he was not accustomed to setting fashion trends.

During high school, Norman did very well and enjoyed participating in debates and was a key member of the debate team. In fact, 1 year they were able to win the state contest. He starred in his Latin class and was class valedictorian when he graduated in January of 1941. He went to the University of Michigan in September of 1941. Initially he thought he would pursue a prelaw degree but also took several classes in engineering. He and a classmate enlisted when it was clear they were going to be drafted. Once in the army he took an aptitude test. A colonel gave him the choice of the infantry, or medicine or dentistry as alternatives. He was quick to select a career as a doctor.

He was sent to Waco, Texas to complete an accelerated premed course, and from there, he went to Vanderbilt in 1945 where he graduated with a medical degree in 1949. While at Vanderbilt, he spent a summer at the Massachusetts General Hospital in 1948. There he was impressed that several surgeons were reading about new operations being performed at the University of Minnesota. The University of Minnesota became a place that he was certain he would apply to for a surgical residency.

He arrived at the University of Minnesota in the summer of 1949. His first 2 years were spent performing general surgery. He was in the Air Force Reserve and was called up in 1951 and spent 2 years in Texas and Louisiana during the Korean Conflict. He returned to the University of Minnesota in 1953 and spent 2 years working toward a PhD. At that time F. John Lewis was his mentor, and his PhD thesis was on hypothermia. His final 2 years at the University of Minnesota were on the clinical wards in general surgery and cardiac surgery. In those times, the surgical resident was usually in the position of a second assistant during a cardiac case. It was at that time that he realized that one of the hardest things about cardiac surgery was getting the opportunity to perform cardiac surgery.

While at the University of Minnesota, he had married Mary Lou Stuurmans, and after receiving his PhD in 1956, he was eager to complete his surgical residency. He asked Dr. Wangensteen when that might be possible. He was asked how many publications he had to his name and replied that there were seven. Dr. Wangensteen thought that he should have a few more before he finished; my father informed Dr. Wangensteen that perhaps reading the papers rather than counting them was a more appropriate way of judging academic performance.

Another episode is well documented in G. Wayne Miller's book about C. Walton Lillehei called, "The King of Hearts" [1]. It occurred on rounds when Dr. Wangensteen thought that a patient was suitable for a second-look operation.

E-mail address: shumw001@umn.edu

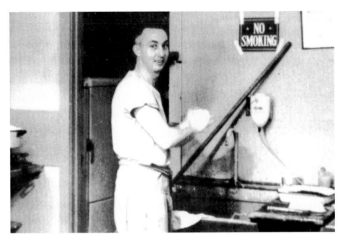

Fig. 1. Norman Shumway scrubs in the dog lab, circa 1960. (*Courtesy of* Sara J. Shumway, MD, Minneapolis, MN.)

The patient herself thought that Dr. Lillehei was Dr. Wangensteen, and despite Dr. Wangensteen's best efforts, she would not believe that he was Dr. Wangensteen. On rounds with Dr. Wangensteen at the time, when Dr. Wangensteen left her room, Dr. Shumway put his arm around him and said, "You know you've got to stop this going around the hospital telling everyone you are Dr. Wangensteen!"

Upon completing the surgical residency in 1957, the Shumways traveled to Santa Barbara, California. There Dr. Shumway joined an older partner in private practice and performed one of the first open-heart operations in California at Cottage Hospital in Santa Barbara. It was successful; however, the combination of the older conservative thoracic surgeon and the younger cardiac surgeon was not a good match; after 6 weeks, Dr. Shumway was fired for what was called "gross insubordination." He interviewed at the University of California, but found a job at Stanford doing primarily research activity as well as performing hemodialysis.

By that time, the Shumway family had grown to include four children, and it was important to have a paying job. While in the laboratory at Stanford, in somewhat rustic conditions, the early work in topical cooling for myocardial preservation as well as heart transplantation took place. Helping him in the laboratory was a young resident surgeon named Richard Lower. Under conditions whereby the roof leaked, and whereby some of the time they were forced to leave to perform dialysis at various places around San Francisco, the situation was less than ideal. They did have funding, however, and they did have plenty of animals as well as plenty of time on their hands. Perhaps this is the ideal setting for the young academic attending.

In 1958, the Stanford Medical School moved to Palo Alto and a large number of the big-city physicians did not accompany this move. Therefore, by default, Norman Shumway became the

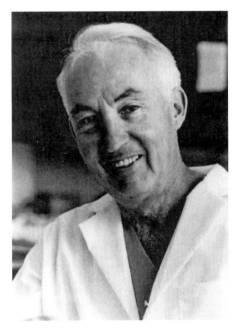

Fig. 2. Norman Shumway, circa 1987. (*Courtesy of* Sara J. Shumway, MD, Minneapolis, MN.)

one and only cardiac surgeon at the Stanford campus. He was told repeatedly that he would be replaced as soon as they could get a big name to come to Stanford. During this period of little clinical work and the slow process of building a clinical program, the laboratory thrived with activities like heart transplants and studies on myocardial protection. In 1960, at the Surgical Forum, Lower presented their work on heart transplantation [2]. It was an early-morning talk, and apparently only the projectionist, the moderator, and Dr. Shumway and Dr. Lower were present. They were hoping for a larger draw. Work continued in the laboratory, and clinical work in congenital heart disease began to surface at the Palo Alto campus. One of the earliest series was on patients who had tetralogy of Fallot. It was found that these patients did better with topical cooling of the heart in the operating room. In fact, Lower, when he took his oral boards in thoracic surgery, spoke of 100 patients undergoing tetralogy of Fallot repairs without a mortality. The examiner thought he was making it up.

It was not until 1967 in a *Journal of American Medical Association* article that Dr. Shumway said the way was paved to perform clinical heart transplantation [3]. This was after a dog named Ralphy had been able to live for a year with another dog's heart. On December 3, 1967, in Groote Schuur Hospital in Cape Town, South Africa, Christiaan Barnard performed the first human heart transplant. The patient lived for 18 days. Barnard had had the opportunity to watch Lower perform a heart transplant on an animal at the Medical College of Virginia, and was able to make arrangements to do the procedure on a human in South Africa without some of the steps felt necessary in the United States. On January 2, 1968, Adrian Kantrowitz performed a heart transplant on an infant who died on the table. That same week Barnard performed his second heart transplant on a dentist named Philip Blaiberg.

It was not until January 6, 1968, that doctors at Stanford University performed the first adult heart transplant in the United States. The patient, Mike Kasperak, lived for 15 days before dying of what Dr. Shumway called "a galaxy of complications." At that time, Dr. Shumway felt that heart transplants should be performed only on patients who were desperately ill and had no other alternative. Some of these patients were so ill that there was already an element of multiorgan

system failure, and that made for a difficult postoperative course. Two years later, it was fairly routine for the patients to at least make it out of the hospital.

In 1970, Dr. Shumway appeared before a Senate subcommittee because various surgeons had called for a moratorium on heart transplantation. This included Michael DeBakey. Frank Church who was a Democratic senator from Idaho was instrumental in allowing doctors at Stanford University to continue to perform heart transplantation. The early 1970s saw a slow increase in the number of heart transplants over a period of time. Approximately a dozen were done on an annual basis until the advent of cyclosporine changed things.

In 1973, the Santa Clara county coroner and the Stanford hospital administrators agreed not to use donors that were the victims of homicide. In September of that year, the Alameda county district attorney called to offer a heart donor at the request of the next of kin. The donor was in Oakland, and the heart was removed at Highland hospital and brought by helicopter to Stanford, and the transplant proceeded. Unfortunately the defense at trial felt that the gunshot victim would have recovered had the surgeons not removed the heart. Fortunately the Harvard panel had convened and the diagnosis of brain death was well established [4]. The judge was able to instruct the jury that the definition of brain death had been respected. The appropriate verdict was reached, and the State of California had a precedent for the legislature to redefine death in terms of brain function. This legal precedent allowed for the use of remote heart procurement.

In 1971, Philip Caves came to Stanford as a British American research fellow. Working in conjunction with Margaret Billingham, an established cardiac pathologist, they developed a technique for and were able to interpret the results of percutaneous transvenous endomyocardial biopsies. His bioptome really revolutionized the way rejection was diagnosed. During the 1970s, only two institutions were doing much in the way of heart transplantation in the United States. These were Lower's group at Medical College of Virginia and Shumway's group at Stanford University.

There were several ongoing projects that continued to improve survival. It was not, however, until the advent of cyclosporine in the late 1970s that survival was good enough to interest other groups in performing heart transplants. It was also in 1978 that Dr. Bruce Reitz began working on heart–lung transplants, which were brought into the clinical arena on March 9, 1981. The patient who received a heart–lung transplant on that day was operated on by Dr. Reitz with Dr. Shumway in his favorite role as first assistant. The patient was able to live 5 years before she died of a problem completely unrelated to her heart–lung transplant. Throughout the late 1960s and early 1970s, Dr. Shumway traveled widely throughout the United States and the world. He functioned as the pied piper of heart transplantation. By the 1980s, he had a well-rehearsed talk on the evolution of heart transplantation.

He took great pride in the progress of his trainees and their contributions to the field. From Wangensteen, he seemed to have taken to heart the idea that professional jealousy was not contributory and a lot more could be accomplished when no one cared who received the credit. He was a great facilitator of other people's ideas at Stanford. He enthusiastically encouraged his fellows to take leadership roles throughout the United States and Europe.

In 1986, he was surprised to learn that he had been made a Vice President of the American Association for Thoracic Society (AATS). He did not realize that this meant that he would then become the President of the AATS. Dr. Sabiston was able to cover for him by having a robot accept the title of Vice President. A year later, his presidential address was very well received. He reviewed Stanford's progress over the years and was quick to give everyone appropriate credit. He was also humorous, and he was especially pleased with the amount of laughter generated.

I believe he would consider his key accomplishment to be:

- Topical cardiac hypothermia [5]
- Auto transplantation of the pulmonic valve into the aorta [6]
- Excision of the mitral valve and replacement with the autologous pulmonic valve [7]
- Congenital heart surgery with early successful series involving repair of tetralogy of Fallot
- Valve replacement with biologic valves
- Orthotopic homotransplantation of the canine heart [8]
- Long-term survival of cardiac homografts in dogs [9]
- Heart transplantation in human
- Diagnosis of cardiac allograft rejection by transvenous endomyocardial biopsy [10]

- Heart–lung transplantation [11]
- Pediatric heart transplantation
- Lobar lung transplantation [12]
- Management and treatment of aortic aneurysms and dissections
- Training of numerous, dedicated cardiovascular surgeons

Professionally I think his only regret was that he did not have the opportunity to take on leadership roles in other surgical societies besides the AATS. I think he felt it was important for him to stay at Stanford and direct the clinical and research activity there. He did travel widely to promote heart transplantation, but did not participate actively in the usual surgical societies.

Dr. Shumway retired from his role as chief of cardiovascular surgery at Stanford University on February 9, 1993. There was an appropriate university-sponsored event. Almost all of his trainees were able to return. During the ensuing 13 years of semiretirement, he continued to operate off and on for 3 more years and enjoyed hearing about other people's cases in a vicarious manner. He enjoyed offering advice, which was asked for frequently. He enjoyed golfing more and continued to travel. His last year of life was complicated by many health issues. He gave it all he had, but the last 6 weeks proved that it was time to move on. Those who know him well are left with lasting memories of good times and multiple quips.

In the operating room, he felt the best thing the surgeon could do under any circumstance was to keep his or her cool. This was a lasting lesson he learned from Walt Lillehei. He had several other sayings that would come up at any appropriate time. These include: "Time will tell. Air rises. The pump is your friend. All bleeding stops. Never quit in a fit of pique. There is plenty of time for sleep on the other side of the grave." He was a good father, friend, and mentor, and he lived a life complete.

References

[1] Wayne Miller G. King of hearts. New York: Times Books, Random House; 2000. p. 207.
[2] Lower RR, Shumway NE. Studies in orthotropic homotransplantations of the canine heart. Surg Forum 1960;11:18–9.
[3] Shumway NE. Way is clear for heart transplant. JAMA 1967;202:31.
[4] Report of the Ad Hoc Committee of the Harvard Medical School to Examine the Definition of Brain

Death. A definition of irreversible coma. JAMA 1968;205:85.

[5] Shumway NE, Lower RR. Topical cardiac hypothermia for extended periods of aortic arrest. Surg Forum 1959;10:563.

[6] Lower RR, Stofer RC, Shumway NE. Autotransplantation of the pulmonic valve into the aorta. J Thorac Cardiovasc Surg 1960;39:680.

[7] Lower RR, Stofer RC, Shumway NE. Total excision of the mitral valve and replacement with the autologous pulmonic valve. J Thorac Cardiovasc Surg 1961;42:696.

[8] Dong E Jr, Hurley EJ, Lower RR, et al. Performance of the heart two years after autotransplantation. Surgery 1964;56:270.

[9] Lower RR, Dong E Jr, Shumway NE. Long-term survival of cardiac homografts. Surgery 1965;58: 110.

[10] Billingham ME, Caves PK, Dong E Jr, et al. Diagnosis of canine orthotropic cardiac allograft rejection by transvenous endomyocardial biopsy. Transplant Proc 1973;5:741.

[11] Reitz BA, Wallwork J, Hunt SA, et al. Heart-lung transplantation: successful therapy for patients with pulmonary vascular disease. N Engl J Med 1982;306:557.

[12] Starnes VA, Lewiston NJ, Luikart H, et al. Current trends in lung transplantation. Lobar transplantation and expanded use of single lungs. J Thorac Cardiovasc Surg 1992;104:1060.

ELSEVIER
SAUNDERS

Heart Failure Clin 3 (2007) 117–120

HEART
FAILURE
CLINICS

A Tribute to Michael E. DeBakey

O.H. Frazier, MD[a,b,*]

[a]Texas Heart Institute at St. Luke's Episcopal Hospital, Houston, TX, USA
[b]Baylor College of Medicine, Houston, TX, USA

Declared a living legend by the United States Library of Congress, Michael Ellis DeBakey has long been one of the world's leading surgical scientists. As a clinician, educator, and researcher, Dr. DeBakey embodies the noble ideas and humanitarian values that characterize the medical profession at its best.

Born in Lake Charles, Louisiana, in 1908, Michael E. DeBakey was the son of Lebanese immigrants who valued education and instilled a love of learning in their children. Because his father owned two pharmacies, Dr. DeBakey was exposed to the medical profession at an early age. Perhaps influenced by this early experience, he decided in his youth to become a doctor.

Medical training

Michael DeBakey earned his bachelor's and medical degrees at Tulane, graduating from medical school in 1932. Dr. DeBakey once told me that one of his activities as a medical student was to help organize the library of Dr. Rudolph Matas, the pioneer of aneurysm surgery. He also helped in translating journal articles into English from French, a language in which Dr. DeBakey was fluent. Also as a medical student, he gained the notice of Dr. Ochsner [1], chairman of the Department of Surgery, who became his mentor. Together, they published many scientific articles. One of these articles was among the first to correlate lung disease with smoking.

During his last year of medical school, Dr. DeBakey [2] developed a small continuous-flow roller pump designed to simplify and improve techniques for blood transfusion. Years later, on a collaborative visit to the laboratory of Dr. John Gibbon, Dr. DeBakey offered a model of his device to assist with the ongoing development of Gibbon's heart–lung machine. In 1953, after successfully performing the first open-heart operation, Dr. Gibbon credited the DeBakey roller pump as a crucial component of his final design.

After receiving his MD degree, Dr. DeBakey completed his internship and surgical residency at Charity Hospital in New Orleans and 2 years of surgical training in Europe (1936–1937) before returning to Tulane University to become an instructor in surgery.

Military service

With the advent of World War II, Dr. DeBakey volunteered for military service and was assigned to the United States surgeon general's office, where he rose to the rank of colonel. During his years of service (1942–1946), he recognized the need for a mobile surgical unit that would allow soldiers to be treated on the combat field. He convinced the surgeon general of the importance of forming what eventually came to be known as Mobile Army Surgical Hospitals (MASH units). For developing these units, Dr. DeBakey was awarded the US Army Legion of Merit in 1945.

While still in military service, Dr. DeBakey recognized that the Army's medical library was one of the finest collections in the world but that it was housed in inadequate facilities. Dr. DeBakey initiated a movement to establish the National Library of Medicine, which was created by

* Texas Heart Institute at St. Luke's Episcopal Hospital, PO Box 20345, MC 2-114A, Houston, TX 77225-0345.

E-mail address: lschwenke@heart.thi.tmc.edu

Congress in 1956. Dr. DeBakey has continued a life-long involvement with the library, serving first as a board member and later as its chairman.

Being especially sensitive to the medical needs of soldiers, Dr. DeBakey also proposed the creation of medical centers designed exclusively for veterans. The first Veterans Administration Hospital was established in Houston in 1949 on the recommendation of Dr. DeBakey. In recognition of his contributions to the welfare of veterans, in 2003 the Michael E. DeBakey Veteran's Administration Medical Center at Houston was named in his honor.

Career at Baylor College of Medicine

In 1948, Dr. DeBakey accepted the position of chairman of the department of Surgery at Baylor University College of Medicine, now Baylor College of Medicine. There, his talent for organizational innovation led to numerous developments. Dr. DeBakey's protean interest and abilities were applied in many areas. As a result of his administrative talents and leadership, by the early 1950s, Baylor had become one of the leading medical schools for surgical innovation. A seminal contribution to this field was Dr. DeBakey's pioneering work in repairing arterial aneurysms with Dacron grafts [3–14]. Nearly every aspect of cardiovascular surgery was influenced by his tireless work ethic and innovative mind. To address the subject of this monograph, however, the remaining comments are confined to Dr. DeBakey's role in the development of mechanical circulatory support devices for advanced heart failure.

Partial and total artificial hearts

The first observation that the work of the heart could be temporarily replaced by a pump, such as the DeBakey roller pump, established the groundwork for mechanical circulatory assistance. Another important observation reported by Dr. DeBakey [15] was the potential for recovery of the failed heart by simple prolongation of cardiopulmonary bypass. These two observations advocated by Dr. DeBakey (ie, the ability of circulatory support to replace heart function and the ability of the heart to recover following "cardiac rest" by mechanical assistance) formed the basis of all subsequent developments in the field.

At Baylor, Dr. DeBakey energetically created a team of the most talented physicians and researchers to aid in the developmental work of cardiac-assist devices. Two of the leading researchers in this field were Dr. William Hall and Dr. Domingo Liotta. As a Baylor student, I had the privilege of working with Dr. Hall and Dr. Liotta, and, in 1965, I wrote a student research paper on cardiac support devices, which was based on my work with these two leaders.

Significant research in this field would have been impossible, however, without government funding, which sustained the development of future cardiac-assist devices. Recognizing this, Dr. DeBakey [16–18] took his message to Washington. In 1963, he spoke before Congress about the need for a total artificial heart, and his testimony was instrumental in persuading the National Institutes of Health to establish the Artificial Heart Program (1964) to support the development of such a device (Fig. 1).

Throughout the 1960s, researchers in the Baylor Surgical Laboratories were known for their leadership in the field of mechanical circulatory support, which was due in part to funding received from the National Institutes of Health. On July 18, 1963, after years of research with animal models, Dr. DeBakey performed the first successful clinical implant of a left ventricular

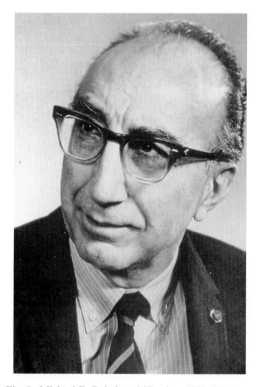

Fig. 1. Michael E. Debakey, MD, circa 1963. (*Courtesy of* O.H. Frazier, MD, Houston, TX.)

assist device (LVAD) in a 42-year-old man suffering from postoperative left ventricular failure. This early device consisted of a double-lumen Silastic and Dacron tube connecting the left atrium with the descending aorta. Using pressure from an external air source, the outer tubing would expand and collapse to create unidirectional flow through the inner blood chamber. Although this pump worked well for 4 days, the patient died of causes unrelated to the technology.

The next pump used was an extracorporeal, hemispherical device with an internal molded diaphragm separating the blood and gas collection chambers. This pneumatically actuated (pressurized CO_2) LVAD was first successfully implanted in a human on August 8, 1966. The patient was a 37-year-old woman who could not be weaned from the heart lung machine following dual valve replacement. The pump provided 10 days of postcardiotomy support before the patient recovered sufficiently for pump explantation; she was a long-term survivor [19].

The design of Dr. DeBakey's left ventricular bypass pump later served as the basis of his first total artificial heart model, created in September of 1968. The pump itself consisted of two separate pumping chambers, made of Dacron-Silastic composite, to replace the right and left ventricles. After removal of all of the heart except the posterior atrial walls, the device was sewn in using cuffs of Dacron fabric. Silastic tubing was brought through the ribs to power both gas chambers, and DeBakey Dacron arterial grafts were used to provide the outflow tracts to the pulmonary artery and ascending aorta. As in the left ventricular bypass pump, the entire blood chamber was lined with Dacron velour fabric to protect the tissue interface.

Since the early 1980s, Dr. DeBakey [20] has devoted much of his energy to the DeBakey VAD (MicroMed Cardiovascular, Inc., Houston, Texas), which he and Dr. George Noon, also of Baylor, developed with the National Aeronautics and Space Administration. One tenth of the size of a traditional LVAD, the DeBakey pump has been implanted in more than 200 patients, including children. Owing to its mechanical simplicity and small size, it is more reliable than earlier devices and can be used in a wider variety of patients.

Honors

In 1965, Dr. DeBakey was featured on the cover of *Time* magazine because of his surgical expertise, teaching ability, and innovative research, particularly on the artificial heart. Over the years, his most prestigious honors have included the American Medical Association Distinguished Service Award (1959), the Albert Lasker Award for Clinical Medical Research (1963), the Presidential Medal of Freedom (1969), the National Medal of Science (1987), inclusion in the Russian Academy of Sciences as the first foreign member (1999), and the Library of Congress Bicentennial Living Legend Award (2000).

Summary

The concept of the ideal, or good, physician has always exerted a powerful hold on the imagination. According to patient surveys [21–23], traits of the ideal physician include not only mastery of the technical elements of care but also confidence, empathy, forthrightness, humaneness, personal interest, respect, thoroughness, courage, prudence, trustworthiness, and honesty. Throughout his career, Dr. DeBakey has exemplified this ideal.

Dr. DeBakey was as stern a taskmaster as I have experienced. He demanded that the patients' well being be the primary goal of medical care. He did not expect difficulties to be overcome without sacrifice or care to be given without compassion. There was no excuse for ineptitude, and mediocrity could only be overcome by diligent work and by utmost application of your talents and experience. Lack of dedication, no matter the personal cost, was never acceptable. Giving up was never voluntary but only an acquiescence to nature's judgment, and quitting was not an option. These were valuable lessons for the care of critically ill patients—lessons that have been guiding principles throughout my career.

Today, at age 98, Dr. DeBakey continues to be an inspiration and a role model, especially for those of us who have known him personally, and I will always be deeply grateful for his mentorship and support.

References

[1] Ochsner A, DeBakey ME. Carcinoma of the lung. Arch Surg 1941;42:209–58.

[2] DeBakey ME. A simple continuous-flow blood transfusion instrument. New Orleans Med Surg J 1934;87:386–9.

[3] DeBakey ME, Cooley DA, Crawford ES, et al. Clinical application of a new flexible knitted Dacron arterial substitute. Am Surg 1958;24:862–9.

[4] DeBakey ME, Cooley DA. Successful resection of aneurysm of thoracic aorta and replacement by graft. JAMA 1953;152:673–6.

[5] DeBakey ME, Cooley DA, Creech O Jr. Surgical considerations of dissecting aneurysms of the aorta. Ann Surg 1955;142:586–612.

[6] DeBakey ME. Successful carotid endarterectomy for cerebrovascular insufficiency. Nineteen-year follow-up. JAMA 1975;233:1083–5.

[7] DeBakey ME, Creech O Jr, Morris GC Jr. Aneurysm of thoracoabdominal aorta involving the celiac, superior mesenteric, and renal arteries. Report of four cases treated by resection and homograft replacement. Ann Surg 1956;144:549–73.

[8] Cooley DA, DeBakey ME. Resection of entire ascending aorta in fusiform aneurysm using cardiac bypass. JAMA 1956;162:1158–9.

[9] DeBakey ME, Crawford ES, Cooley DA, et al. Successful resection of fusiform aneurysm of aortic arch with replacement by homograft. Surg Gynecol Obstet 1957;105:657–64.

[10] DeBakey ME, Crawford ES, Morris GC Jr, et al. Patch graft angioplasty in vascular surgery. J Cardiovasc Surg 1962;3:106–41.

[11] DeBakey ME, Cooley DA. Surgical treatment of aneurysm of abdominal aorta by resection and restoration of continuity with homograft. Surg Gynecol Obstet 1953;97:257–66.

[12] Cooley DA, DeBakey ME. Surgical considerations of excisional therapy for aortic aneurysms. Surgery 1953;34:1005–20.

[13] DeBakey ME, Cooley DA. Treatment of aneurysms of the aorta by resection and restoration of continuity with aortic homograft. Angiology 1954;5:251–4.

[14] Crawford ES, DeBakey ME, Cooley DA. Clinical use of synthetic arterial substitutes in three hundred seventeen patients. AMA Arch Surg 1958;76: 261–70.

[15] DeBakey ME, Liotta D, Hall CW. Left-heart bypass using an implantable blood pump. In: Mechanical Devices to Assist the Failing Heart. Presented at the National Research Council (U.S.). Committee on Trauma. Washington, DC, September 9–10, 1964.

[16] DeBakey ME. The odyssey of the artificial heart. Artif Organs 2000;24:405–11.

[17] DeBakey ME. Development of a ventricular assist device. Artif Organs 1997;21:1149–53.

[18] DeBakey ME, Liotta D, Hall CW. Prospects for and implications of the artificial heart. J Rehabil 1966;32: 106–7.

[19] DeBakey ME. Left ventricular bypass pump for cardiac assistance. Am J Cardiol 1971;27:3–11.

[20] Wieselthaler GM, Schima H, Hiesmayr M, et al. First clinical experience with the DeBakey VAD continuous-axial-flow pump for bridge to transplantation. Circulation 2000;101:356–9.

[21] Bendapudi NM, Berry LL, Frey KA, et al. Patients' perspectives on ideal physician behaviors. Mayo Clin Proc 2006;61:338–44.

[22] Li JT. The quality of caring. Mayo Clin Proc 2006; 81:294–6.

[23] Pellegrino ED. Professionalism, profession and the virtues of the good physician. Mt Sinai J Med 2002;69:378–84.

ELSEVIER
SAUNDERS

Heart Failure Clin 3 (2007) 121–137

HEART
FAILURE
CLINICS

Expectations of Surgeons from an Imager

Hind Rahmouni, MD, Martin St. John Sutton, MD, FRCP*

University of Pennsylvania Medical Center, Philadelphia, PA, USA

Congestive heart failure is a clinical syndrome characterized by fatigue, shortness of breath, exercise intolerance, and fluid retention with lower extremity and/or pulmonary edema. There is an estimated 25 to 30 million patients who have heart failure worldwide. Heart failure is primarily a disease of the elderly, and the prevalence of chronic heart failure increases with advancing age. Currently, chronic heart failure is the most common hospital discharge diagnosis in patients over the age of 65 years. Thus, as the population ages, the management of heart failure will become more frequent and of even greater importance. The management of patients who have heart failure is challenging, and the mortality with medical therapy alone is high. Although the ideal treatment for heart failure is cardiac transplantation, this therapy is limited by a chronic shortage of donor hearts. Currently, the mainstay of heart failure treatment is pharmacologic and includes angiotensin converting enzyme inhibitors, angiotensin receptor blockers, β-adrenergic receptor blockers, aldosterone receptor antagonists, diuretics, and digitalis. However, surgery is becoming increasingly important with valve repair/replacement, ventricular assist devices, and epicardial restraints.

Systolic versus diastolic heart failure

Heart failure may be systolic due to abnormal myocardial excitation–contraction coupling or diastolic due to abnormal relaxation and increased

myocardial passive stiffness. Between 30% and 50% of all patients presenting with heart failure have diastolic heart failure (left ventricle [LV] ejection fraction $\geq$ 50%). Diastolic heart failure was initially believed to be a rare and benign condition, but the annual mortality from diastolic heart failure ranges from 5% to 15%, and admission rate for recurrent heart failure is 50% within the first 6 months [1–4]. The remaining 50% to 70% of patients present with systolic heart failure that is clinically indistinguishable from diastolic heart failure. It is important to identify patients who have systolic heart failure because they may be eligible for surgical therapy. The important information in systolic heart failure for the surgeon from an imaging perspective is the reliable and reproducible assessment of LV size, architecture, and function, because these are the strongest predictors of clinical outcome following cardiac surgery. We therefore focus attention on systolic heart failure and how imaging modalities can optimize the type and timing of surgical treatment.

Assessment of left ventricle function

There are several different imaging modalities available for qualitative and quantitative assessment of LV function: echocardiography, nuclear imaging, contrast angiography, cardiac magnetic resonance (CMR) imaging, and CT. CMR is considered the gold standard for estimation of LV volumes, mass, and function (LV ejection fraction [LVEF]), because of its high spatial and temporal resolution and its ability to quantify LV volume from tomographic slices without geometric assumptions regarding LV cavity shape (Fig. 1). However, echocardiography is more commonly used than CMR in clinical practice for assessment of LV volumes and function because of its wider availability. Echocardiography

* Corresponding author. Division of Cardiology, University of Pennsylvania Medical Center, 3400 Spruce Street, Philadelphia, PA 19104.

E-mail address: suttonm@mail.med.upenn.edu (M. St. John Sutton).

1551-7136/07/$ - see front matter © 2007 Elsevier Inc. All rights reserved.
doi:10.1016/j.hfc.2007.04.002

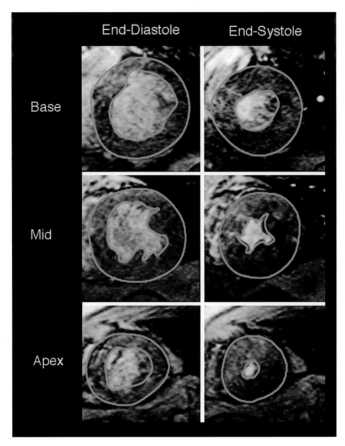

Fig. 1. Calculation of LV volumes by cardiac MRI. A series of stacked short axis images are analyzed and contoured using a semiautomated edge-detection algorithm. Cardiac MRI is especially useful for deformed ventricles because no geometric assumptions are necessary for quantitative measurements of ventricular volumes and mass. (*Courtesy of* V.A. Ferrari, Philadelphia, PA.)

is noninvasive, provides good spatial and temporal resolution, and is inexpensive. The American Society of Echocardiography recommends biplane Simpson's rule method for calculating LV volumes from an apical four-chamber and apical two-chamber view, or from a single apical two-chamber view [5]. LV volumes determined by echocardiography correlate closely with contrast angiography and CMR [6]. Assessment of LV volumes by echocardiography relies heavily on the expertise of the interpreter identifying endocardial borders, which is labor-intensive, time-consuming, and costly.

There are several new echo technologies such as use of echo contrast or new computer software applications based on artificial intelligence and speckle tracking that facilitate automated identification of the endocardium and almost instantaneously quantify LV volumes and ejection fraction.

Although LVEF is widely used to assess global LV function, LVEF is really a measure of chamber function rather than myocardial function because it is load-dependant. When loading conditions are abnormal (eg, in valvular heart disease), LVEF may suggest normal LV chamber function, even when intrinsic myocardial function is severely depressed. This apparent disconnect has clinical implications in aortic and mitral regurgitation whereby reliance on LVEF may erroneously delay surgical intervention with valve repair or replacement.

Indications and preoperative assessment for surgery

What the surgeon needs to know
from the imager about acute myocardial infarction

Echocardiography is an important tool in acute myocardial infarction for determining infarct size and location, detecting mechanical complications (acute mitral regurgitation from papillary muscle rupture, ventricular septal defect, cardiogenic shock), and stratifying risk. Surgical intervention in acute myocardial infarction has become increasingly common; what the surgeon wants to know from the imager is the presence of specific mechanical complications, assessment of the hemodynamics and LV function, and the indications and timing of surgery. The 2003 American College of Cardiology (ACC)/American Heart Association (AHA)/ASE guidelines [7] recommend the use of echocardiography for the assessment of mechanical complications after acute myocardial infarction as a class I indication.

Ventricular septal defect

Ventricular septal defect (VSD) is a severe complication of acute myocardial infarction with an incidence of 0.4% to 0.7% in the era of thrombolytic therapy [8]. Risk factors for VSD include age over 60 years, female sex, first myocardial infarction, and hypertension. VSD is more common with large anterior infarcts without collateral blood flow. VSD associated with inferior infarction tends to occur toward the base of the heart, making surgical access more difficult, so that the prognosis is worse for inferior than anterior infarct VSDs. The average time to development of a VSD is 5 days, and the defect may range in size from 1 to 10 mm. The size of VSD and the consequent hemodynamics significantly influence the mortality. Infarction VSDs are optimally treated surgically, and the definitive diagnosis must be established preoperatively. Echocardiography usually enables direct visualization of the defect and the adjacent akinesis or dyskinesis (Fig. 2). Color Doppler demonstrates the high-velocity turbulent jet traversing the septal defect. The continuous wave Doppler demonstrates a systolic gradient across the VSD. Transesophageal echocardiography may be useful in cases in which the transthoracic images are nondiagnostic especially in patients requiring mechanical ventilation support.

The surgeon also needs to know the exact location of the entrance and exit of the infarct VSD because closure of VSD is invariably achieved through the right ventricle by way of the tricuspid valve. Other prerequisites for surgical closure include the size of the shunt (Qp/Qs), VSD location, pulmonary arterial systolic pressure, ventricular function, and the degree of heart failure, all of which can be readily obtained by Doppler echocardiography.

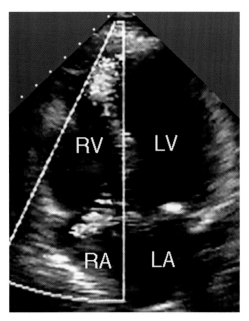

Fig. 2. Transthoracic apical four-chamber view of a patient who had antero septal myocardial infarction and apical ventricular septal defect shown by color flow Doppler.

Acute severe mitral regurgitation

Acute MR following acute myocardial infarction portends a poor prognosis and usually occurs in single coronary artery disease. Severe regurgitation can result from acute rupture of a papillary muscle head, which usually involves the inferoposterior papillary muscle. Acute MR may also result from acute ischemic dysfunction of the papillary muscle and adjacent LV wall without rupture. The presence of severe MR and the etiologic mechanisms must be ascertained and the severity of regurgitation quantified before corrective surgery is contemplated. Echo diagnosis may be difficult with transthoracic imaging, and often transesophageal Doppler echocardiographic is necessary to establish the diagnosis. Severity of MR can usually be adequately semiquantitated using graded Doppler color flow mapping (0 = none/trivial, 1 = mild, 2 = moderate, 3 = severe).

Cardiogenic shock

Echocardiography can detect early infarct expansion and aneurysm formation that occurs after anterior myocardial infarctions. Infarct expansion is the stimulus for progressive LV dilatation and remodeling to heart failure. Unopposed

LV dilatation and aneurysm formation may result in cardiogenic shock, thrombus formation, stroke, and LV rupture. Before remedial surgical intervention, crucial information required by the surgeon is an accurate assessment of LV size and function, and the presence of mechanical defects (MR or VSD). Before left ventricular assist device (LVAD) placement for cardiogenic shock, significant apical thrombosis and aortic regurgitation needs to be excluded to avoid stroke risk and LVAD malfunction, respectively.

What the surgeon needs to know from the imager about indications for surgery and preoperative assessment in chronic coronary disease/post infarction

Coronary artery disease (CAD) is the major cause (70%) of heart failure [9]. Prognosis of patients who have ischemic heart failure and medical therapy alone is poor. Comparison of medical versus surgical therapy for CAD has excluded patients who have an LVEF less than 35% [10]. However, improvements in surgical techniques have shown that coronary bypass surgery may be performed with acceptable mortality, even in patients who have severe ventricular dysfunction [11]. A significant subgroup of patients who have heart failure and underlying CAD has reversible LV dysfunction following revascularization. In patients who have depressed LV function, the poorer the LV function, the greater is the likelihood of improvement post coronary artery bypass grafting (CABG) surgery. Although the relative benefit is similar to the other patients, the absolute benefit is greater because of the high-risk profile of these patients [12]. Thus, identification of subsets of patients who have CAD and LV dysfunction who benefit from revascularization is important to optimize patient outcome.

Coronary angiography is still considered the reference standard for the diagnosis of coronary artery disease. However, there are new techniques that provide diagnostic information about proximal occlusive CAD, especially the 64-slice CT coronary angiography and electron beam CT.

Contrast coronary angiography provides crucial information to the surgeon regarding the location and severity of stenoses, the number of coronary arteries involved, and global and regional left ventricular function before CABG surgery. One additional important question posed by the surgeon before CABG is the viability of the region of myocardium to be revascularized.

Viability

Myocardial viability is extremely important to establish before surgical revascularization because it predicts the clinical outcome and postop LV function. Viable myocardium is characterized by several attributes, including cell membrane integrity, intact mitochondria, preserved glucose metabolism, intact resting p erfusion, and inotropic reserve. The absence of myocardial shortening is not reliable as an indicator of viability because metabolic activity can be present in hibernating or stunned myocardium. There are several techniques that predict myocardial viability, some of which are impractical, unavailable, or confined to quaternary medical centers.

F-18 fluorodeoxyglucose positron emission tomography. Positron emission tomography (PET) is considered the gold standard for assessment of myocardial viability [13] by assessing the homogeneity of regional myocardial glucose metabolism. The magnitude of improvement in heart failure symptoms after revascularization in patients who have LV dysfunction correlates with the preoperative extent of F-18 fluorodeoxyglucose (FDG) "mismatch."

Dobutamine stress echocardiography. Dobutamine augments myocardial contractility at low doses and increases heart rate and peripheral vasodilatation at higher doses. In ischemic regions, there is a biphasic response. Low doses of dobutamine augment contractility, but higher doses decrease myocardial shortening resulting in regional wall motion abnormalities. In patients who have CAD and severe LV dysfunction who demonstrated myocardial viability during dobutamine echocardiography, revascularization improved survival compared with medical therapy [14]. Recent advances in echo technology, such as echo contrast, harmonic imaging, speckle tracking, and artificial intelligence that enhance endocardial border definition, may improve diagnostic accuracy in detecting viability.

Nuclear imaging. In myocardial single photon emission computed tomography (SPECT) with Tc-99 m, the regional functional recovery following revascularization increases in proportion to Tc-99 m sestamibi uptake. In the segments with greater than 55% maximal uptake, the likelihood of functional recovery is greater than 70%. However, there are two different conditions that may result in a mild to moderate decrease in uptake of radionuclide flow tracers: (1) chronically decreased blood flow in hibernating viable myocardium, and

(2) a nontransmural infarct supplied by either a patent or occluded proximal coronary vessel. Although revascularization will likely be beneficial in the former situation, it will not be likely to improve regional function in the latter. Thallium (Tl-201) nuclear imaging is an energy-dependent process that requires intact cell membranes. The presence of a reversible perfusion defect and/or preserved Tl-201 uptake on the 3- to 4-hour redistribution images is an important sign of regional viability. The mean sensitivity in predicting functional recovery is 86%. However, specificity is only 59%, indicating that in approximately 40% of patients who have delayed thallium-201 uptake, there was no evidence of regional functional recovery following revascularization. In a study of patients who had heart failure, Marin-Neto and colleagues [15] showed that thallium SPECT with reinjection yields information regarding regional myocardial viability that is similar to that provided by PET in patients who have severe as well as moderate LV dysfunction. However, there is discordance in over 20% of regions manifesting severe irreversible thallium defects in patients who have severely reduced LV function.

Cardiac magnetic resonance. The spatial resolution of CMR enables differentiation of subendocardial versus transmural myocardial viability. A new CMR method to assess myocardial viability is the detection of "delayed hyperenhancement." Following MRI contrast injection, T1- and T2-weighted images demonstrate decreased signal intensity in regions of myocardial scar and also in areas of resting ischemia (ie, hibernating myocardium). In delayed images, myocardial scar tissue accumulates contrast (delayed hyperenhancement), whereas resting ischemia does not. If less than 25% of the thickness of a myocardial wall demonstrates delayed hyperenhancement, wall motion will improve following revascularization. CMR hyperenhancement correlates with F-18 FDG PET data [16].

All of the four methods previously described can provide the surgeon with information about the viability of regions of myocardial ischemia that he/she planned to revascularize.

What the surgeon needs to know about ischemic MR

Chronic ischemic MR is an MR occurring more than 1 week after myocardial infarction with: (1) one or more left ventricular segmental wall motion abnormalities, (2) significant coronary disease in the territory supplying the wall motion abnormality, and (3) structurally normal mitral valve (MV) leaflets and chordae tendinae. The third criterion is particularly important because it excludes patients who have organic MR and associated coronary artery disease.

Ischemic MR occurs in approximately 20% of patients after myocardial infarction and in 56% of patients who have congestive heart failure caused by ischemic or nonischemic cardiomyopathy [17]. There is a graded independent association between the severity of ischemic MR and the development of heart failure after myocardial infarction. Even mild ischemic MR is associated with an increase in the risk of heart failure [18].

The ischemic insult results in LV remodeling toward a more spherical shape with new wall motion abnormalities. These changes lead to annular dilatation and subvalvular distortion that prevents the mitral leaflets from coapting normally during systole (Fig. 3) [19,20]. Elucidation of the pathogenesis of ischemic MR relates largely to alterations in ventricular geometry and function. This finding has led investigators to question surgical techniques that only address the mitral valve annulus [21] because annuloplasty alone fails in 20% to 30% of patients who have ichemic MR [22].

Ischemic mitral regurgitation is often clinically silent and should be systematically evaluated by imaging. Standard color Doppler imaging is a highly sensitive method to detect even mild degrees of ischemic mitral regurgitation. A unique advantage of echocardiography is that it accurately quantifies the severity of mitral regurgitation by the effective regurgitant orifice area and calculates the regurgitant volume [23]. Congestive heart failure is independently determined by larger effective regurgitant orifice area (Fig. 4) [24]. In some patients who have exertional dyspnea out of proportion to their resting systolic dysfunction or MR, exercise echocardiography can reveal the true severity of what might otherwise be considered mild MR. Peteiro and colleagues [25] demonstrated that exercise echocardiography has a higher prognostic value compared with resting echocardiography. An exercise-induced increase in effective regurgitant orifice area greater than 13 mm^2 is an independent predictor of cardiac death [26].

Three-dimensional (3D) transthoracic echocardiography (TTE) and transesophageal echocardiography (TEE) are new and promising tools to

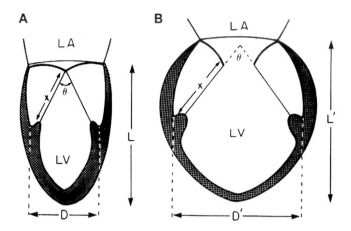

Fig. 3. Schematic demonstrating a possible mechanism of mitral regurgitation. (*A, B*) Left ventricular dilatation due to volume overload results in the left ventricle becoming more spherical. The mitral valve ring circumference increases. The angle subtended by the papillary muscles to the mitral annulus increases, but there is no elongation of the mitral valve leaflets or chordae, which results in incomplete cusp coaptation and mitral regurgitation.

assess the anatomy of the mitral valve (Fig. 5). New parameters can be measured using 3D: mitral valve tenting volume, the nonplanar angle (Fig. 6), annulus circumference, annulus area, and 3D commissural length. 3D has a higher sensitivity than TEE in detecting commissural and bileaflet defects [27]. It is also a promising method for the direct measurement of the effective regurgitant orifice area. 3D echocardiography overcomes the limitations of the proximal isovelocity surface area and is also unaffected by orifice shape [28]. Preoperative increased mitral annular diameter, tethering area, and MR grade

were associated with repair failure in ischemic MR [29]. The LV may continue to remodel and dilate, rendering initial repair ineffective [30].

Detection of thrombus

TTE is the standard procedure for detection of LV thrombosis with a sensitivity ranging from 92% to 95% and a specificity of 95% assuming good image quality. However, in routine clinical cardiologic practice, poor image quality occurs in approximately 10% to 20% of patients, particularly at the apex where thrombus is most likely to form. Contrast echocardiography can be used to

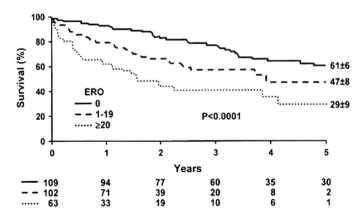

Fig. 4. Effect of severity of ischemic MR, assessed by effective regurgitant orifice area (ERO) of at least 20 mm^2 or less than 20 mm^2 on survival. (*From* Grigioni F, Enriquez-Sarano M, Zehr KJ, Bailey KR, Tajik AJ. Ischemic mitral regurgitation: long-term outcome and prognostic implications with quantitative Doppler assessment. Circulation 2001;103:1762; with permission.)

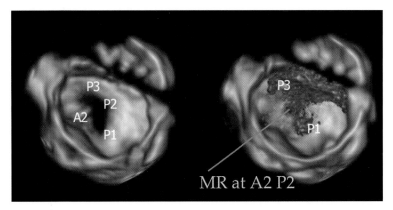

Fig. 5. Mitral valve visualized by three-dimensional transesophageal echocardiography (*right*) and with color Doppler (*left*) showing the anatomy of the mitral regurgitation.

improve visualization of the blood/tissue interface and detection of the endocardial borders. TEE cannot be considered a reference technique for LV thrombosis assessment because of its limitation to adequately visualize the LV apex. Detection of thrombus is extremely important before surgical LVAD placement to avoid propagation of thrombus into the systemic circulation causing stroke.

Detection of pulmonary hypertension
The presence of pulmonary hypertension increases morbidity and mortality postoperatively in patients who have cardiomyopathies, valvular heart disease, and coronary artery disease. Pulmonary artery systolic pressure can be determined noninvasively by Doppler echocardiography using the modified Bernoulli equation. The peak velocity of tricuspid regurgitation reveals the systolic right ventricular to right atrial pressure gradient ($P = 4V^2$), and the right atrial pressure, estimated from the respiratory change in vena caval diameter, is then added to the gradient to obtain the pulmonary artery pressure.

What the surgeon needs to know from the imager about indications for surgery and preoperative assessment in chronic valvular heart diseases

Degenerative MR
Quantitative grading of asymptomatic mitral regurgitation is a powerful predictor of the clinical outcome [31]. Patients who have an effective regurgitant orifice greater than 40 mm^2 should be considered for cardiac surgery. Cardiac surgery in these patients was independently associated with improved survival (adjusted risk ratio, 0.28).

Preoperative assessment of MV anatomy is essential for planning surgical repair/replacement of degenerative MV disease with and without leaflet prolapse. Although two-dimensional TTE and TEE provide precise information regarding MV anatomy, 3D TTE and 3D TEE increases the understanding of more complex abnormalities of MV apparatus and improves individual scallop identification. Pepi and colleagues [32] demonstrated that

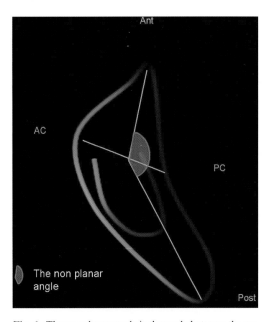

Fig. 6. The nonplanar angle is the angle between the anterior leaflet plane and the posterior leaflet plane at the commissural diameter. It is proportional to the degree of flatness of the mitral annulus and the loss of the saddle shape. AC, anterior commissure; PC, posterior commissure.

3D TTE and 3D TEE are superior for accurate localization and identification of MV pathology in comparison with the two-dimensional echo methods. Real-time 3D echo allows precise localization of the diseased mitral commissures and individual scallops. Improvements in acquisition and reconstruction times will provide the surgeon with dynamic detailed continuous images that will enable more sophisticated and durable surgical repair techniques.

The ACC/AHA guidelines criteria for severe MR are the same for ischemic MR and degenerative MR and consist of a regurgitant volume of at least 60 mL per beat, a regurgitant fraction of at least 50%, and a regurgitant orifice area of at least 0.4 cm^2 (Table 1).

Aortic stenosis

Aortic stenosis (AS) is the most common valvular heart disease resulting in valve replacement [33]. There is no alternative to surgery when the patient presents with symptoms of heart failure due to severe aortic stenosis (class I indication) [7]. Imaging techniques and especially echocardiography play a vital role in surgical aortic valve replacement during the preoperative, intraoperative, and postoperative periods. Echocardiography also allows identification of associated lesions, such as

Table 1

Criteria for severe valvular disease according to the American College of Cardiology/American Heart Association 2006 guidelines

Indicator	Severe sortic stenosis
Jet velocity	> than 4.0 m/s
Mean gradient	> 40 mm Hg
Valve area	< 1.0 cm^2
Valve area index	< 0.6 cm^2/m^2
Severe aortic regurgitation	
Qualitative	
Angiographic grade; 3–4+	
Color Doppler jet width; central jet, width > 65% LVOT	
Doppler vena contracta width; > 0.6 cm	
Quantitative (cath or echo)	
Regurgitant volume; ≥ 60 mL/beat	
Regurgitant fraction; ≥ 50%	
Regurgitant orifice; area ≥ 0.30 cm^2	
Additional essential criteria	
Left ventricular size; increased	
Severe mitral regurgitation	
Qualitative	
Angiographic grade; 3–4+	
Color Doppler jet area; large central MR jet (area >40% of LA area) or with a wall impinging jet of any size, swirling in LA	
Doppler vena contracta width; > 0.7 cm	
Quantitative (cath or echo)	
Regurgitant volume; ≥ 60 mL/beat	
Regurgitant fraction; ≥ 50%	
Regurgitant orifice area; ≥ 0.40 cm^2	
Additional essential criteria	
Left atrial size; enlarged	
Left ventricular size; enlarged	

Abbreviations: LA, left atrium; LVOT, left ventricular outflow tract.

Data from American College of Cardiology/American Heart Association Task Force on Practice Guidelines, Society of Cardiovascular Anesthesiologists, Society for Cardiovascular Angiography and Interventions, Society of Thoracic Surgeons, Bonow RO, Carabello BA, Kanu C, et al. ACC/AHA 2006 guidelines for the management of patients with valvular heart disease: a report of the American College of Cardiology/American Heart Association Task Force on Practice Guidelines (writing committee to revise the 1998 Guidelines for the Management of Patients With Valvular Heart Disease): developed in collaboration with the Society of Cardiovascular Anesthesiologists: endorsed by the Society for Cardiovascular Angiography and Interventions and the Society of Thoracic Surgeons. Circulation 2006;114:E84–231.

concomitant mitral and tricuspid valve disease, concomitant CAD, and ascending aortic aneurysm; and/or left-sided obstructive lesions, such as coarctation that are associated with bicuspid aortic stenosis that may require surgical attention.

The surgeon wants to know from the imager the pathoetiology of the AS and the size of the aortic root to avoid inserting too small a prosthesis and causing patient/prosthesis mismatch identified by elevated postoperative transvalve systolic gradients (Fig. 7). The surgeon also wants to be certain that the patient who has heart failure and AS does indeed have severe AS and not simply a calcified valve and heart failure due to coronary artery disease or coexistent cardiomyopathy.

Quantification of severity: three echocardiographic parameters are used routinely to assess the severity of AS, blood flow velocity, pressure gradient, and valve area (see Table 1). AS is considered severe if velocity is greater than 4 m/s, gradient is greater than 40 mm Hg, and valve area is less than 1 cm^2.

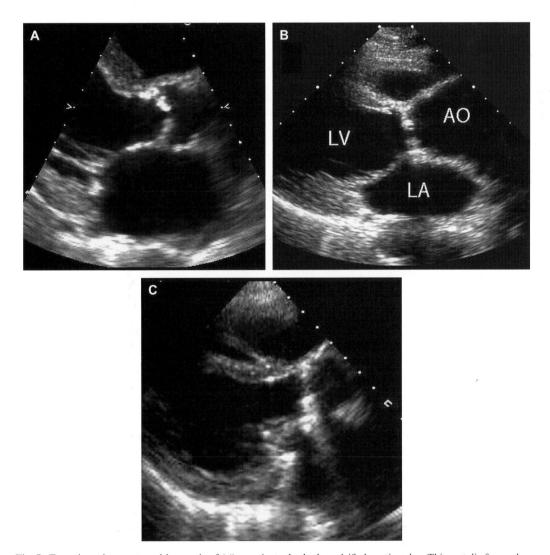

Fig. 7. Transthoracic parasternal long axis of (*A*) a patient who had a calcified aortic valve. This systolic frame shows a limited opening of the aortic valve of (*B*) a patient who had aortic stenosis and an aneurysmal aortic root. (*C*) Patient prosthesis mismatch due to replacement of too small an aortic prosthesis. There is also a prosthesis in the mitral position. AO, aortic root; LA, left atrium.

Aortic valve orifice area is less dependent of LV function than is the transvalvular gradient. Aortic velocity is the most reproducible and is the strongest predictor of clinical outcome [34]. Echocardiographic methods have largely replaced catheterization for the routine evaluation of AS. Catheterization plays a confirmatory role and for assessment of coexistent coronary artery disease.

Special situations. In patients who have low cardiac output, it is crucial to differentiate severe aortic stenosis complicated by systolic heart failure from mild to moderate aortic stenosis associated with systolic heart failure of a different etiology. In the former situation, surgery is required, whereas in the latter situation, surgery is not indicated. In selected patients who have low-flow/low-gradient AS and LV dysfunction, it is useful to measure the transvalvular pressure gradient and calculate valve area during a baseline state and during exercise or low-dose pharmacologic (dobutamine) stress (class IIa indication) [7]. In patients who have AS and poor LV function, it may be difficult to determine the predominant condition, and AVA may increase with increased stroke volume. Dobutamine stress echo may be used to establish whether AVA increases significantly with dobutamine; if so, severe AS is not present. If the transaortic gradient increases with increased stroke volume, the AS is severe.

TEE is important for preoperative and perioperative sizing of the aortic root for homograft placement. Sizing of the aortic root and pulmonary valve is also essential to the successful completion of the Ross procedure.

Aortic regurgitation

In the Western world, severe aortic regurgitation (AR) is usually due either to congenital diseases (bicuspid valve) or degenerative conditions (such as annuloaortic ectasia), which typically present in the fourth to sixth decades. In rare cases, aortic regurgitation is acute, caused by endocarditis or aortic dissection. Patients who have severe aortic regurgitation have higher morbidity and mortality than the general population [35]; and within 10 years of the diagnosis of severe AR, heart failure occurs in approximately half the patients, most of whom require aortic-valve replacement. The optimal treatment of chronic severe AR and heart failure is aortic valve replacement, even if the LV is severely dilated and the LVEF is low. The surgeon needs to be sure from an imaging perspective that there is severe AR and that the abnormal LV architecture and function are directly related to the AR and whether other valve pathology, CAD, or ascending aortic aneurysms need to be addressed.

Transthoracic Doppler echocardiography is the main imaging modality for diagnosing and assessing the severity of aortic regurgitation. Color flow Doppler is exquisitely sensitive for detecting even mild subclinical AR. Severe AR is defined by the ACC/AHA 2006 guidelines (see Table 1) as a regurgitant volume of at least 60 mL, a regurgitant fraction of at least 50%, a regurgitant orifice area of at least 0.3 cm^2, a central jet width greater than 65% left ventricular outflow tract, and a "vena contracta" (width of the regurgitant flow stream at the orifice) of at least 0.6 cm with a high specificity for measurements that are at least 0.7 cm [7,36].

What the surgeon needs to know from the imager about indications for surgery and preoperative assessment in congenital heart disease

Imaging in congenital heart disease is beyond the scope of this manuscript; but it must provide the surgeon with an accurate description of intracardiac anatomy. This is achieved in complex cyanotic congenital heart disease by adhering to a scanning protocol that systematically determines atrial situs, atrioventricular, and ventricular arterial connections. Atrial and ventricular function and the presence of intra- or extracardiac shunts are also evaluated. This information can be obtained and analyzed by two-dimensional and real-time 3D echocardiography, CMR, and also 3D CT.

Intraoperative echocardiography

TEE imaging is used by the surgeon in the operating room as a perioperative diagnostic tool rather than a monitoring device. TEE often reveals new and unexpected pathology that may impact upon surgical and anesthetic therapy.

Pre- and postevaluation of function and monitoring of ischemia

TEE allows assessment of global and regional LV function. It can detect new regional wall motion abnormalities, associated with ischemia, and is frequently used for intraventricular monitoring of LV ischemia.

Pre- and postprocedure evaluation of MR

Intraoperative TEE is a useful tool in MR surgery because it enables the surgeon to understand the precise mechanism of valvular dysfunction. This assessment needs to be performed dynamically with the heart beating and the ventricle maintaining a full cardiac output at a normal blood pressure. Anesthetic induction and inotropic agents can substantially reduce the severity of MR. It is not sufficient to examine the competence of the valve on cardiopulmonary bypass with the heart arrested. Once the repair has been completed and the patient separated from bypass, the adequacy of the repair can be assessed by TEE before the chest is closed. Therefore, remedial repair work can be undertaken to the valve without recourse to a subsequent operation.

Additional, unanticipated intraoperative findings

Intraoperative TEE is valuable in uncovering significant abnormalities that have been overlooked during the preoperative assessment. Kneeshaw [37] showed that intraoperative TEE changed the surgical management in 26% of patients with a change in the procedure itself in 20% of patients.

Evaluation of the aorta for the clamping site

The most important predictor of brain injury, transient ischemic attack, or stroke in the perioperative period is a severely atherosclerotic and/or calcific/porcelain ascending aorta before or during the bypass operation [12]. Perioperative embolism from aortic plaque is responsible for almost one third of strokes after CABG. Preoperative noninvasive imaging to identify high-risk patients can be obtained with CT, TEE, and CMR. The surgeon wants to know from the imager about the presence and location of atheromatous ulcers, plaques, and adherent thrombus in the ascending aorta to select appropriately safe cross-clamp sites [38] to minimize stroke risk.

What the surgeon wants to know about postoperative assessment

Early complications

Pericardial effusion and tamponade

Cardiac tamponade is an uncommon but life-threatening complication following cardiac surgery. The diagnosis of pericardial tamponade may be difficult to establish early postop by TTE when the patient is lying flat and ventilated, so that TEE is often required for definitive diagnosis. Additionally, a pericardial clot may be highly localized and difficult to detect. In pericardial tamponade, echocardiography shows diastolic collapse of the right ventricle, late diastolic inversion of the right atrium, and inferior cava plethora with blunted respiratory variation. Right atrial collapse during diastole is a sensitive but not specific sign of tamponade. Inversion of the right atrium for more than one third of the R-R interval is considered sensitive (94%) and specific (100%) for a hemodynamically significant pericardial effusion. Doppler findings consistent with pericardial tamponade include: delayed mitral valve opening, marked respiratory variation, and reciprocal changes in mitral and tricuspid valve inflow Doppler velocity signals.

Endocarditis

Infective endocarditis with vegetations, fistulae, and valve abscess can occur with native and prosthetic valves. TEE is superior to TTE for the detection of valvular vegetation; ring abscesses; and other complications, particularly with mitral prostheses. Accurate early diagnosis of endocarditis is critically important to avoid complications. Indications for surgery in endocarditis include abscess cavities, avulsion of the valves and large (>10 mm) mobile vegetations on account of their propensity to embolize, all of which are assessable by echo. These are usually readily detectable with TTE, but if image quality is suboptimal or doubt remains as to the secure diagnosis, TEE should be performed without hesitation (Table 2).

Early valves complications

Structural failure is common in bioprosthetic valves at long-term follow-up, especially in young patients. Paravalvular leaks early after surgery can be detected with intraoperative TEE or postoperative TTE. The reported incidence ranges from 18% to 48% of patients who have a mitral or aortic prosthesis; the majority of leaks are trivial or mild and do not progress over a 2- to 5-year follow-up period. In contrast, late development of new paravalvular leaks should suggest endocarditis or structural failure and initiate an intense search for a causative micro-organism.

Table 2

Indications for surgery in endocarditis according to the American College of Cardiology/American Heart Association 2006 guidelines

Surgery for native valve endocarditis	
Class I	1. Patients who have acute infective endocarditis who present with valve stenosis or regurgitation resulting in heart failure
	2. Patients who have acute infective endocarditis who present with aortic regurgitation or mitral regurgitation with hemodynamic evidence of elevated LV end-diastolic or left atrial pressures (eg, premature closure of MV with AR, rapid decelerating MR signal by continuous-wave Doppler, or moderate or severe pulmonary hypertension)
	3. In patients who have infective endocarditis by fungal or other highly resistant organisms
	4. Patients who have infective endocarditis complicated by heart block, annular aortic abscess, or destructive penetrating lesions
Class IIa	Patients who have infective endocarditis who present with recurrent emboli and persistent vegetations despite appropriate antibiotic therapy
Class IIb	Patients who have infective endocarditis who present with mobile vegetations in excess of 10 mm with or without emboli
Surgery for prosthetic valve endocarditis	
Class I	1. Consultation with a cardiac surgeon is indicated for patients who have infective endocarditis of a prosthetic valve
	2. Patients who present with heart failure
	3. Patients who present with dehiscence evidenced by cine fluoroscopy or echocardiography
	4. Patients who present with evidence of increasing obstruction or worsening regurgitation
	5. Patients who present with complications (eg, abscess formation)
Class IIa	1. Patients who present with evidence of persistent bacteremia or recurrent emboli despite appropriate antibiotic treatment
	2. Patients who present with relapsing infection
Class III	Surgery is indicated for patients who have uncomplicated infective endocarditis of a prosthetic valve caused by first infection with a sensitive organism

Data from American College of Cardiology/American Heart Association Task Force on Practice Guidelines, Society of Cardiovascular Anesthesiologists, Society for Cardiovascular Angiography and Interventions, Society of Thoracic Surgeons, Bonow RO, Carabello BA, Kanu C, et al. ACC/AHA 2006 guidelines for the management of patients with valvular heart disease: a report of the American College of Cardiology/American Heart Association Task Force on Practice Guidelines (writing committee to revise the 1998 Guidelines for the Management of Patients With Valvular Heart Disease): developed in collaboration with the Society of Cardiovascular Anesthesiologists: endorsed by the Society for Cardiovascular Angiography and Interventions and the Society of Thoracic Surgeons. Circulation 2006;114:E84–231.

Late complications

Repeat coronary artery bypass grafting

Repeat coronary artery bypass grafting (redo-CABG) in patients who have ischemic cardiomyopathy is associated with high perioperative risk and worse long-term outcome compared with patients who have first CABG [39]. This risk is even higher in patients who have LV dysfunction. However, viability testing was not performed in these studies reporting poor outcome of patients undergoing redo-CABG. Rizzello and colleagues [40] demonstrated that patients who have ischemic cardiomyopathy and a substantial amount of viable myocardium undergoing redo-CABG benefit from revascularization in terms of improvement in LVEF and heart failure symptoms. These improvements are similar to those observed in patients who have first CABG. Therefore, the

selection of patients for redo-CABG should be based on the presence of viable myocardium.

Late valves complications

The overall incidence of complications in appropriately managed patients is approximately 3% per year. The ACC/AHA guideline [7] has a class I recommendation for echocardiography for assessing prosthetic heart valve complications. An echocardiogram should be obtained at baseline ideally before hospital discharge for every patient (class I recommendation). This baseline echocardiogram is extremely important because it serves to establish the "identity card" of the prosthetic valve for further comparison during follow-up. This study will document the stability of the valve, the presence and extent of valvular or paravalvular regurgitation, and the transvalvular pressure gradients. The "normal gradient" across a prosthetic valve depends upon the type, size, and position of the prosthesis as well as the cardiac output; guidelines are available for the acceptable range of Doppler gradients encountered in properly functioning valves. The ACC/AHA guidelines [7] actually do not recommend an annual routine echocardiography in patients who have mechanical valves or during the first 5 years with bioprosthetic valves unless there is a change in clinical status. However patients who have bioprosthetic valves may be considered for annual echocardiography after the first 5 years in the absence of a change in clinical status (IIb). An echocardiography should be performed anytime if there is a change in clinical status.

The most common prosthesis complications are: extrinsic interference of function (pannus, thrombus, vegetation) resulting in obstruction or regurgitation, perivalvular leak, strut fracture and component escape, leaflet tear of bioprosthesis, and leaflet calcification/stenosis of bioprosthesis.

Because of its more anterior position, aortic prosthesis can be imaged more efficiently by TTE than mitral prosthesis. Assessment of mechanical prosthetic malfunction is more difficult with TTE because acoustic shadowing caused by the prosthetic material may limit transthoracic visualization of prosthetic leaflets, vegetations, abscesses, and thrombi. TEE should be performed when TTE does not clearly identify the site and/or

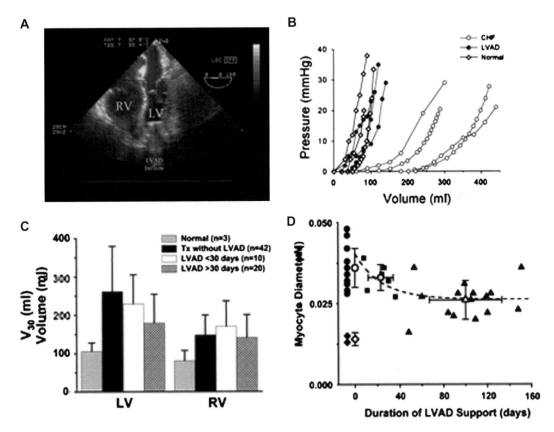

Fig. 8. (A) Transesophageal echocardiogram of patient who had HeartMate vented electric LVAD showing volume unloading of left atrium and LV, whereas right-sided chambers remain volume loaded. (B) Ex vivo LV end-diastolic pressure–volume relations (EDPVR) measured from normal hearts, failing hearts, and end-stage failing hearts supported with LVAD explanted at time of transplantation. (C) With heart size indexed by V30, volume on EDPVR at which pressure is 30 mm Hg, it is seen that LV reverse structural remodeling occurs and is more prominent after than before 30 days of support. In contrast, there is no significant reverse remodeling of right ventricle. (D) Time course of regression of cellular hypertrophy during LVAD support. (From Mancini D, Burkhoff D. Mechanical device-based methods of managing and treating heart failure. Circulation 2005;112:444; with permission.)

mechanism of malfunction of a prosthetic valve. TEE imaging of the prosthesis enables direct inspection of the valve leaflets, which should be imaged through multiple cardiac cycles. Prosthetic malfunction can be divided in those cases with predominant obstruction in which the Doppler mean and peak gradient are severely increased, and those with predominant regurgitation in which transvalvular velocities are normal or minimally increased.

Semisurgical procedures

Left ventricular assist devices

LVADs are assuming a greater role in the care of patients who have end-stage heart failure. Initially, these devices were only used as a bridge to transplant, but recently patients who have advanced heart failure have recovered normal LV function [41], opening a broad application for LVAD as a bridge to recovery rather than a bridge to transplant. Ventricular-assist devices have also been placed for destination therapy in patients who have intractable heart failure who are not candidates for heart transplantation. LVADs target LV remodeling that is a major culprit in the development of heart failure. Prolonged unloading of the LV relieves the chronically elevated wall stress and starts the process of reverse remodeling, which is the main goal of heart failure treatment (Fig. 8).

Echocardiographic screening for significant aortic regurgitation and LV apical thrombus before insertion is important to avoid sucking blood from the aorta and systemic embolization, respectively, during insertion of the LV cannula (Fig. 9). LVADs may provide pulsatile or nonpulsatile flow; the settings of the LVAD pump are routinely evaluated by Doppler echocardiography over a range of flows and correlate closely with LVAD flow rates. When there is divergence between the two estimates of flow, the Doppler flow is invariably lower suggesting partial obstruction of the LV outlet usually by thrombus forming within or protruding into the LV apical cannula [42]. Partial occlusion of the LV outlet cannula is confirmed by the presence of flow acceleration by color flow Doppler map and a gradient across the LV apical outflow cannula (Fig. 10).

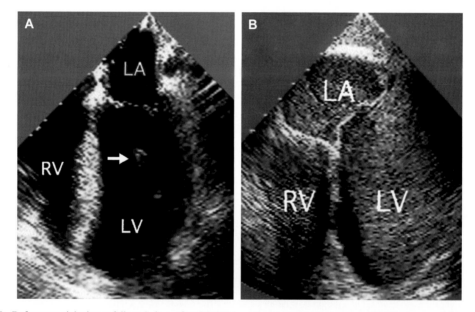

Fig. 9. Refractory right heart failure 3 days after LVAD insertion, requiring emergent RVAD placement in a patient who had persistently low LVAD flows. (*A*) Intraoperative TEE shows a small mobile thrombus in the LV in the four-chamber view. Failure to regain consciousness and progressive hypotension led to a repeat TEE 2 days later. (*B*) This transesophageal view demonstrates almost complete cardiac thrombosis. The normal geometry of the heart is distorted by the thrombus. The patient died from stroke and multiorgan failure on the following day. LA, left atrium; RV, right ventricle. (*From* Reilly MP, Wiegers SE, Cucchiara AJ, et al. Frequency, risk factors, and clinical outcomes of left ventricular assist device-associated ventricular thrombus. Am J Cardiol 2000;86:1158; with permission.)

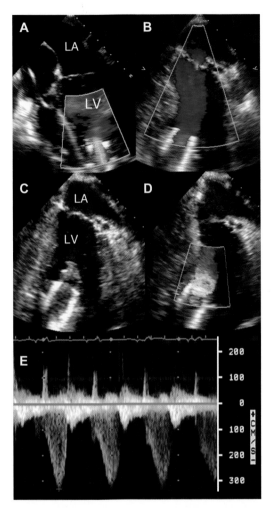

Fig. 10. Transesophageal views of a patient who had a left ventricular assist device. (*A, B*) The canula is visible at the LV apex. (*C, D*) A thrombus can be seen on LVAD canula with a color flow Doppler showing the obstruction. Spectral Doppler showing a systolic gradient across the LVAD draining canula indicating partial obstruction by thrombus. (*From* Reilly MP, Wiegers SE, Cucchiara AJ, et al. Frequency, risk factors, and clinical outcomes of left ventricular assist device-associated ventricular thrombus. Am J Cardiol 2000;86:1158; with permission.)

Restraint devices

An alternative method proposed to decrease wall stress and to reduce reverse remodeling is by passive epicardial restraint devices. Animal studies showed that LV dilatation and remodeling could be prevented, and LV function preserved by placing a nondistensible material on the epicardium overlying a subsequent myocardial infarction [43]. The first device that underwent clinical trial was an epicardial mesh that enveloped both ventricles and was tested in patients who had New York Heart Association (NYHA) class III/IV, LV dilatation, and end-stage LV dysfunction. Doppler echocardiograms showed that the device prevented progressive LV enlargement without constriction and in a proportion of patients was associated with symptomatic improvement and increased ejection fraction [44]. Two further clinical trials are currently in progress in patients who have NYHA class III/IV systolic heart failure using quantitative serial echocardiography and change in LV volumes as end-points. The results of these on-going clinical trials using Doppler echocardiographic end-points will determine whether these devices will have a major role in the treatment of chronic systolic heart failure.

Summary

In the last decade, we have witnessed an extraordinary development of new cardiac imaging techniques. Some are already in routine use while other promising techniques, such as 3D and intracardiac echocardiography, are still taking their first steps in clinical applications and have not yet revealed all their potential. Heart failure surgery is also evolving rapidly toward less-invasive procedures with the introduction of video-assisted robotic valve repair/replacement surgery, percutaneous delivery of epicardial restraint devices, mitral edge-to-edge clips, coronary sinus mitral annuloplasty rings, and stem cell therapy. These rapid developments are challenging for the imager and the surgeon and mandate a close collaboration between the two disciplines to minimize surgical risk and improve the outcome of patients who have heart failure.

References

[1] Vasan RS, Larson MG, Benjamin EJ, et al. Congestive heart failure in subjects with normal versus reduced left ventricular ejection fraction: prevalence and mortality in a population-based cohort. J Am Coll Cardiol 1999;33:1948–55.

[2] Chen HH, Lainchbury JG, Senni M, et al. Diastolic heart failure in the community: clinical profile, natural history, therapy, and impact of proposed diagnostic criteria. J Card Fail 2002;8:279–87.

[3] Redfield MM, Jacobsen SJ, Burnett JC Jr, et al. Burden of systolic and diastolic ventricular dysfunction in the community: appreciating the scope of the heart failure epidemic. JAMA 2003;289:194–202.

[4] Dauterman KW, Go AS, Rowell R, et al. Congestive heart failure with preserved systolic function in a statewide sample of community hospitals. J Card Fail 2001;7:221–8.

[5] Lang RM, Bierig M, Devereux RB, et al. Chamber Quantification Writing Group, American Society of Echocardiography's Guidelines and Standards Committee, European Association of Echocardiography. Recommendations for chamber quantification: a report from the American Society of Echocardiography's Guidelines and Standards Committee and the Chamber Quantification Writing Group, developed in conjunction with the European Association of Echocardiography, a branch of the European Society of Cardiology. J Am Soc Echocardiogr 2005;18:1440–63.

[6] Darasz KH, Underwood SR, Bayliss J, et al. Measurement of left ventricular volume after anterior myocardial infarction: comparison of magnetic resonance imaging, echocardiography, and radionuclide ventriculography. Int J Cardiovasc Imaging 2002; 18:135–42.

[7] Bonow RO, Carabello BA, Kanu C, et al. American College of Cardiology/American Heart Association Task Force on Practice Guidelines, Society of Cardiovascular Anesthesiologists, Society for Cardiovascular Angiography and Interventions, Society of Thoracic Surgeons. ACC/AHA 2006 guidelines for the management of patients with valvular heart disease: a report of the American College of Cardiology/American Heart Association Task Force on Practice Guidelines (writing committee to revise the 1998 Guidelines for the Management of Patients With Valvular Heart Disease): developed in collaboration with the Society of Cardiovascular Anesthesiologists: endorsed by the Society for Cardiovascular Angiography and Interventions and the Society of Thoracic Surgeons. Circulation 2006;114:E84–231.

[8] Birnbaum Y, Wagner GS, Gates KB, et al. Clinical and electrocardiographic variables associated with increased risk of ventricular septal defect in acute anterior myocardial infarction. Am J Cardiol 2000;86: 830–4.

[9] Bonow RO, Dilsizian V. Thallium 201 for assessment of myocardial viability. Semin Nucl Med 1991;21:230–41.

[10] Rahimtoola SH. A perspective on the three large multicenter randomized clinical trials of coronary bypass surgery for chronic stable angina. Circulation 1985;72:V123–35.

[11] Elefteriades JA, Tolis G Jr, Levi E, et al. Coronary artery bypass grafting in severe left ventricular dysfunction: excellent survival with improved ejection fraction and functional state. J Am Coll Cardiol 1993;22:1411–7.

[12] Eagle KA, Guyton RA, Davidoff R, et al. American College of Cardiology, American Heart Association. ACC/AHA 2004 guideline update for coronary artery bypass graft surgery: a report of the American College of Cardiology/American Heart Association Task Force on Practice Guidelines (Committee to Update the 1999 Guidelines for Coronary Artery Bypass Graft Surgery). Circulation 2004;110:E340–437.

[13] Ghesani M, Depuey EG, Rozanski A. Role of F-18 FDG positron emission tomography (PET) in the assessment of myocardial viability. Echocardiography 2005;22:165–77.

[14] Afridi I, Grayburn PA, Panza JA, et al. Myocardial viability during dobutamine echocardiography predicts survival in patients with coronary artery disease and severe left ventricular systolic dysfunction. J Am Coll Cardiol 1998;32:921–6.

[15] Marin-Neto JA, Dilsizian V, Arrighi JA, et al. Thallium scintigraphy compared with 18F-fluorodeoxyglucose positron emission tomography for assessing myocardial viability in patients with moderate versus severe left ventricular dysfunction. Am J Cardiol 1998;82:1001–7.

[16] Klein C, Nekolla SG, Bengel FM, et al. Assessment of myocardial viability with contrast-enhanced magnetic resonance imaging: comparison with positron emission tomography. Circulation 2002;105:162–7.

[17] Trichon BH, Felker GM, Shaw LK, et al. Relation of frequency and severity of mitral regurgitation to survival among patients with left ventricular systolic dysfunction and heart failure. Am J Cardiol 2003;91: 538–43.

[18] Aronson D, Goldsher N, Zukermann R, et al. Ischemic mitral regurgitation and risk of heart failure after myocardial infarction. Arch Intern Med 2006; 166:2362–8.

[19] De Simone R, Wolf I, Hoda R, et al. Three-dimensional assessment of left ventricular geometry and annular dilatation provides new mechanistic insights into the surgical correction of ischemic mitral regurgitation. Thorac Cardiovasc Surg 2006; 54:452–8.

[20] Kaul S, Spotnitz WD, Glasheen WP, et al. Mechanism of ischemic mitral regurgitation. An experimental evaluation. Circulation 1991;84:2167–80.

[21] Levine RA, Schwammenthal E. Ischemic mitral regurgitation on the threshold of a solution: from paradoxes to unifying concepts. Circulation 2005;112: 745–58.

[22] Tahta SA, Oury JH, Maxwell JM, et al. Outcome after mitral valve repair for functional ischemic mitral regurgitation. J Heart Valve Dis 2002;11:11–8 [discussion: 18–9].

[23] Bursi F, Enriquez-Sarano M, Jacobsen SJ, et al. Mitral regurgitation after myocardial infarction: a review. Am J Med 2006;119:103–12.

[24] Grigioni F, Detaint D, Avierinos JF, et al. Contribution of ischemic mitral regurgitation to congestive heart failure after myocardial infarction. J Am Coll Cardiol 2005;45:260–7.

[25] Peteiro J, Monserrrat L, Bouzas A, et al. Prognostic value of mitral regurgitation assessment during

exercise echocardiography in patients with known or suspected coronary artery disease. J Am Soc Echocardiogr 2006;19:1229–37.

[26] Lancellotti P, Lebrun F, Pierard LA. Determinants of exercise-induced changes in mitral regurgitation in patients with coronary artery disease and left ventricular dysfunction. J Am Coll Cardiol 2003;42: 1921–8.

[27] Muller S, Muller L, Laufer G, et al. Comparison of three-dimensional imaging to transesophageal echocardiography for preoperative evaluation in mitral valve prolapse. Am J Cardiol 2006;98:243–8.

[28] Iwakura K, Ito H, Kawano S, et al. Comparison of orifice area by transthoracic three-dimensional Doppler echocardiography versus proximal isovelocity surface area (PISA) method for assessment of mitral regurgitation. Am J Cardiol 2006;97: 1630–7.

[29] Kongsaerepong V, Shiota M, Gillinov AM, et al. Echocardiographic predictors of successful versus unsuccessful mitral valve repair in ischemic mitral regurgitation. Am J Cardiol 2006;98:504–8.

[30] Hung J, Papakostas L, Tahta SA, et al. Mechanism of recurrent ischemic mitral regurgitation after annuloplasty: continued LV remodeling as a moving target. Circulation 2004;110:II85–90.

[31] Enriquez-Sarano M, Avierinos JF, Messika-Zeitoun D, et al. Quantitative determinants of the outcome of asymptomatic mitral regurgitation. N Engl J Med 2005;352:875–83.

[32] Pepi M, Tamborini G, Maltagliati A, et al. Head-to-head comparison of two- and three-dimensional transthoracic and transesophageal echocardiography in the localization of mitral valve prolapse. J Am Coll Cardiol 2006;48:2524–30.

[33] Selzer A. Changing aspects of the natural history of valvular aortic stenosis. N Engl J Med 1987;317: 91–8.

[34] Otto CM. Valvular aortic stenosis: disease severity and timing of intervention. J Am Coll Cardiol 2006;47:2141–51.

[35] Dujardin KS, Enriquez-Sarano M, Schaff HV, et al. Mortality and morbidity of aortic regurgitation in clinical practice. A long-term follow-up study. Circulation 1999;99:1851–7.

[36] Tribouilloy CM, Enriquez-Sarano M, Bailey KR, et al. Assessment of severity of aortic regurgitation using the width of the vena contracta: a clinical color Doppler imaging study. Circulation 2000;102: 558–64.

[37] Kneeshaw JD. Transoesophageal echocardiography (TOE) in the operating room. Br J Anaesth 2006;97: 77–84.

[38] Hartman GS, Peterson J, Konstadt SN, et al. High reproducibility in the interpretation of intraoperative transesophageal echocardiographic evaluation of aortic atheromatous disease. Anesth Analg 1996;82:539–43.

[39] Weintraub WS, Jones EL, Craver JM, et al. In-hospital and long-term outcome after reoperative coronary artery bypass graft surgery. Circulation 1995; 92:II50–7.

[40] Rizzello V, Poldermans D, Schinkel AF, et al. Outcome after redo-CABG in patients with ischemic cardiomyopathy and viable myocardium. Heart 2007;93:221–5.

[41] Birks EJ, Tansley PD, Hardy J, et al. Left ventricular assist device and drug therapy for the reversal of heart failure. N Engl J Med 2006; 355:1873–84.

[42] Reilly MP, Wiegers SE, Cucchiara AJ, et al. Frequency, risk factors, and clinical outcomes of left ventricular assist device-associated ventricular thrombus. Am J Cardiol 2000;86:1156–9.

[43] Kelley ST, Malekan R, Gorman JH 3rd, et al. Restraining infarct expansion preserves left ventricular geometry and function after acute anteroapical infarction. Circulation 1999;99:135–42.

[44] Blom AS, Mukherjee R, Pilla JJ, et al. Cardiac support device modifies left ventricular geometry and myocardial structure after myocardial infarction. Circulation 2005;112:1274–83.

ELSEVIER
SAUNDERS

Heart Failure Clin 3 (2007) 139–157

**HEART
FAILURE
CLINICS**

Surgery for Heart Failure: Now Something for Everyone?

Stephen Westaby, MS, PhD, FRCS*

Oxford Heart Centre, John Radcliffe Hospital, Headington Oxford, UK

The year 2007 marks the 50th anniversary of two major advances destined to become pivotal in the treatment of heart failure. In 1957 Charles Bailey reported a small series of left ventricular aneurysm resections performed by side clamping of the dyskinetic scar and suture without cardiopulmonary bypass. Performed with low mortality, the operation provided immediate symptomatic relief from breathlessness [1]. The same year, Walton Lillehei and Vincent Gott used direct electrical stimulation of the myocardium to save a 3-year-old child who had tetralogy of Fallot and surgically induced complete heart block [2]. This procedure was the landmark beginning of cardiac pacing (Fig. 1).

For the past 50 years cardiac surgery has been in a continuous state of flux. In congenital heart disease palliative techniques have given way to corrective operations using cardiopulmonary bypass. Rheumatic valve disease has virtually disappeared with the widespread use of antibiotics. Coronary artery bypass surgery (CABG) is in recession with the hugely successful refinement of percutaneous balloon angioplasty and stents. In turn coronary intervention rates will fall because of public health initiatives on diet and smoking together with the widespread use of statins. Stent graft technology now benefits many who would otherwise require extensive high-risk thoracoabdominal aortic surgery. Total artificial hearts have given way to left ventricular assist devices, and pulsatile blood pumps are superceded by miniaturized continuous flow devices. In the same way

that enthusiasm for prosthetic heart valves has waned in favor of valve repair techniques, reconstruction of the failing heart is, for most patients, a more realistic alternative than committal to a transplant waiting list.

Nontransplant heart failure surgery is an expanding field at a time when medical treatment and cardiac resynchronization therapy have recognized limits. Although donor hearts can be supplied to only to a tiny minority of patients who have heart failure, other surgical options may soon provide symptomatic relief for the majority. The demand for treatment emerges from an increasingly elderly heart failure population with greater expectations because of well-publicized medical advances and rapidly evolving technology [3]. The revolution in functional cardiac imaging by three-dimensional echocardiography, magnetic resonance, or contrast-enhanced computerized tomography has provided a much better understanding of the anatomy and pathophysiology of heart failure. The failing heart beats at more than 120,000 beats per day, pumping more than 6,000 L of blood against an increased systemic and pulmonary afterload. As the heart dilates, wall tension, myocardial energy, and oxygen consumption increase. Subendocardial blood flow is diminished in response. It is logical that a pharmacologically or mechanically unloaded heart has the chance for recovery [4]. It is certain that the remodeled and unsupported heart does not. Left ventricular restoration surgery is predicated on the well-defined relationship between cardiac shape, volume, and function (Fig. 2) [5]. Equally, the recent remarkable developments in blood pump bioengineering provide an alternative approach and a platform on which to base genetic or stem cell therapies [6].

* Oxford Heart Centre, John Radcliffe Hospital, Headley Way, Headington, Oxford OX3 9DU, United Kingdom.

E-mail address: stephen.westaby@orh.nhs.uk

1551-7136/07/$ - see front matter © 2007 Published by Elsevier Inc.
doi:10.1016/j.hfc.2007.04.003

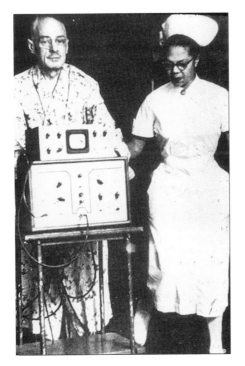

Fig. 1. Cardiac pacing in the late 1950s.

What constitutes the heart failure population?

Congestive heart failure is the final common pathway for many diseases that affect the myocardium (Table 1). Advanced heart failure is defined by symptoms that limit daily activity despite attempted maximum medical therapy (New York Heart Association [NYHA] Functional Class III or IV, or Stage D) [7]. Different clinical conditions predominate in different parts of the world. Although coronary artery disease accounts for more than 65% of cases in North America and Europe (Fig. 3), Chagas disease assumes greater significance for populations with shorter life expectancy in South America. In the Italian SEOSI study 70% of patients had previous myocardial infarction, whereas 15% had hypertensive heart disease [8]. Idiopathic dilated cardiomyopathy and valvular heart disease together accounted for the remaining 15%. Less well understood is that virtually half of heart failure patients have well-preserved left ventricular ejection fraction (LVEF) [9]. From a 15-year experience of heart failure admissions to the Mayo Clinic, Owan and colleagues [10] showed 47% of patients to have preserved left ventricular systolic function (LVEF >50%, mean 61%). Moreover, the diastolic dysfunction group had a similarly dismal prognosis with 29% mortality in 1 year and 65% by 5 years. Clearly LVEF alone is a poor predictor of clinical disability and survival [11].

Heart failure symptoms stem from two main pathophysiologic processes, which can be addressed surgically. Raised left ventricular end diastolic pressure (LVEDP) and impaired filling properties cause pulmonary congestion and breathlessness, whereas decreased systemic blood flow triggers the vascular, cytokine, and humoral

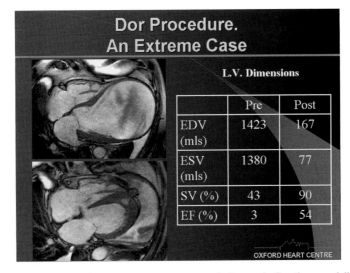

Fig. 2. Left ventricular restoration surgery: an extreme case before and after the remodeling operation.

Table 1
Classification of cardiomyopathies

Inflammatory heart disease	Secondary cardiomyopathy
Viral myocarditis	Endocrine
Idiopathic myocarditis	Rheumatologic
Giant cell myocarditis	Nutritional
Sarcoidosis	Toxic
Eosinophilic myocarditis (hypersensitivity)	Metabolic
Infectious	Inherited
Lyme disease	Neuromuscular disorders
Human immunodeficiency virus	X-linked
Chagas disease	Mitochondrial
Peripartum	Familial dilated cardiomyopathy
Extramyocardial cardiomyopathy	Storage diseases
	Disorders of cardiac energy metabolism
Coronary artery disease	Tachycardia-induced cardiomyopathy
Valvular heart disease	Hemochromatosis
Congenital cardiac anomalies	Amyloidosis
Hypertension	Neoplastic

responses that cause salt and water retention and fatigue. Logically the treatment of this combination depends on an increase in cardiac output and reduction in LVEDP.

Systolic heart failure results from adverse remodeling of the left ventricle in response to a stimulus (myocardial infarction, virus, toxin, and so forth) (Fig. 4). The term "left ventricular remodeling" describes the cardiovascular compensatory mechanism for an acute loss in

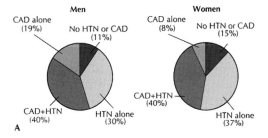

Fig. 3. The epidemiology of heart failure in North America with specific reference to hypertension (HTN) and coronary artery disease (CAD). (*Data from* the Framingham Study.)

myocardial contractile function (Fig. 5) [12,13]. With an increase in LVEDP the chamber dilates to a more spherical shape. Initially this process proves beneficial through the Frank-Starling mechanism because the chamber enlarges to maintain stroke volume even though LVEF falls. Soon dilatation has a progressively detrimental effect because of increased wall tension (La Place law) and impaired subendocardial blood flow. Heart failure progression is characterized by changes in the morphology of the myocyte (enlargement), altered genetic expression to fetal type, and bioenergetic decline with impaired force generation [12]. Disruption of the collagen matrix decreases force transmission, whereas cardiac dyssynchrony results in force wasting. Atrial and ventricular dysrhythmias and intermittent ischemic events compound the problem. Ventricular dilatation eventually causes mitral regurgitation through altered left ventricular geometry, papillary muscle dysfunction, and annular dilatation (Fig. 6a, b) [14]. Progressive volume overload contributes to left ventricular enlargement and worsened mitral regurgitation with decreased survival. Increased chamber sphericity and the onset of mitral regurgitation are important markers of poor prognosis with 1-year mortality between 54% and 70% [15].

For patients who have ischemia the relationship between myocardial infarct size and mortality is clearly defined (Table 2) [16]. If more than 20% of the ventricular circumference is dyskinetic or akinetic, the remaining cavity dilates to preserve stroke volume. When more than 40% of the myocardial circumference is impaired the normal left ventricular end systolic volume index (LVESVI) of 25 mL/m^2 increases to greater than 60 mL/m^2, and elevated wall tension causes progressive left ventricular failure. Hypertrophy of nonischemic segments is a compensatory mechanism for elevated wall stress but increases the potential for dysrhythmia. Myocyte hypertrophy causes prolongation of the action potential and alterations in key sarcolemmal channels and currents that contribute to action potential repolarization [17]. The delayed rectifier current, which is directly responsible for cell repolarization, is reduced in myocyte hypertrophy and is associated with prolongation of the action potential. This prolongation may allow early depolarization and create a reentry circuit promoting dysrhythmia. The Na+/K+ adenosine triphosphatase (ATPase) is also altered in heart failure and may contribute to a more positive and unstable resting potential.

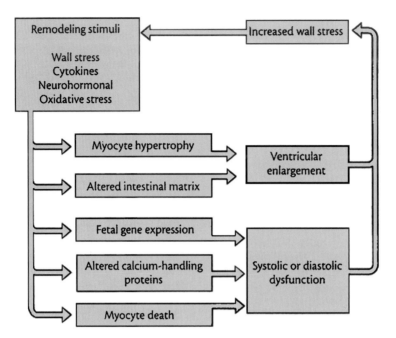

Fig. 4. Cellular and myocardial responses to remodeling stimuli including myocardial wall stress, cytokines, neuroendocrine signals, oxidative stress, and signaling peptides. The myocyte and interstitial matrix changes first normalize wall stress but at the expense of ventricular compliance and function. The net result is further impairment of pump function, escalating wall stress, and a vicious cycle progressing to heart failure.

When the LVESVI exceeds 100 mL/m^2 with LVEF less than 30%, the 5-year survival is around 50% [18]. In this situation most patients have symptomatic congestive heart failure. From the CASS Registry, 5-year survival for patients who had LVEF less than 25% was 41% with medical treatment and 62% with CABG [19]. This finding provided clear evidence at an early stage that surgery could influence the natural history of ischemic heart failure. The benefit of revascularization was an improvement in the contractility of stunned or hibernating myocardium in 60% to 70% of cases as long as the LVESVI remained less than 100 mL/m^2. A critical mass of reversibly ischemic myocardium must be present to achieve global improvement in LV function [20]. No wall motion recovery occurs following revascularization when greater than 50% of myocardial wall thickness is composed of scar tissue [21]. Epicardial salvage by thrombolysis during myocardial infarction thus may not preserve contractility if endocardial necrosis causes scar formation. Patients who have heart failure without reversible ischemia or with LVESVI greater than 100 mL/m^2 do not have improved outlook with revascularization alone and CABG carries substantial mortality risk [22].

The goal of medical and surgical treatment is to delay or arrest progression of the remodeling process. Observational and therapeutic studies show medical treatment to be more successful for nonischemic heart failure than ischemic [23]. In randomized trials with ACE inhibitors, beta-blockers, vasodilators, or milrinone, mortality in the placebo group was consistently 3% to 11% higher for patients who had ischemia [24–26]. This rate translated into 41% 5-year mortality for patients who had ischemia versus 31% for those who did not have ischemia.

Ventricular restoration surgery

Although the addendum "something for everyone" may seem overly optimistic, a systemic review of heart failure interventions suggests that operations and devices are continuously emerging to provide symptomatic relief and improve survival. Fig. 7 considers the heart failure population according to whether there are lesions amenable to conventional surgery, potentially recoverable myocardial disease, or essentially no target lesion or recoverable myocardium. In this last worse-case scenario cardiac replacement or lifetime circulatory support are still feasible.

A

Mechanisms of remodelling in response to myocardial infarction

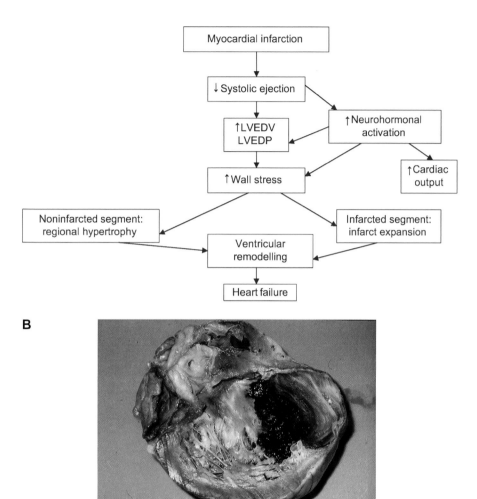

Fig. 5. (*A*) Mechanisms of remodeling in response to myocardial infarction with progression depending on the extent of infarction (Table 2). (*B*) Autopsy specimen of an unoperated extensively remodeled heart, which caused death by congestive heart failure. Surgical ventricular restoration aims to prevent progression to this stage.

Ischemic cardiomyopathy is a heterogeneous condition. Impairment of left ventricular systolic function may be the result of myocardial scar, stunning, or hibernation, and is commonly a combination of these entities within the same heart [27]. The components of postinfarction ventricular remodeling include infarct expansion, myocardial hypertrophy, and global dilatation resulting in a more spherical contour (see Fig. 6). The workload of myocardium remote from the akinetic or dyskinetic area is increased by the dysfunctional changes. Increased wall stress causes lengthening

and thinning of the LV walls through lateral slippage of myocardial planes. Changes in ventricular geometry, wall tension, and filling pressures combine to increase the metabolic requirements of nonischemic myocardium. Abnormalities of diastolic function can also be demonstrated during stress in most patients who have extensive coronary disease. These are manifested by reduced peak left ventricular filling rate and increased time to peak filling rate. Hypoxia impairs relaxation of the papillary muscles during early diastole because this is an active energy-dependent

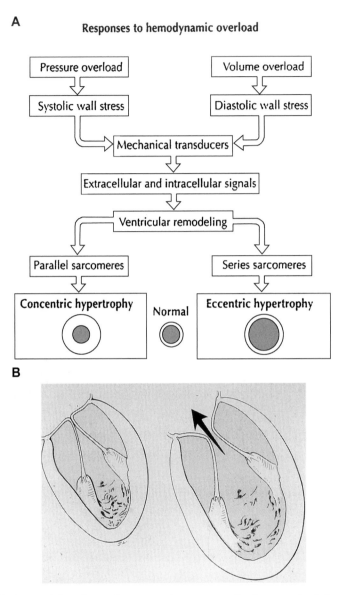

Fig. 6. (*A*) Morphologic remodeling changes in response to pressure and volume overload. In pressure overload (eg, aortic stenosis, hypertension, coarctation of the aorta) increased systolic wall stress leads to parallel addition of sarcomeres and widening of the myocyte. This leads to concentric hypertrophy and diastolic heart failure. In volume overload attributable to regurgitant valve disease there is increased ventricular volume. This leads to a series addition of sarcomeres and lengthening of the myocyte causing "eccentric" hypertrophy and systolic heart failure. (*B*) Development of mitral regurgitation.

process. Abnormalities of systolic and diastolic LV function may be sufficiently severe during stress to cause elevated LVEDP with dyspnea and angina during ischemic episodes. Some patients have increased LVEDP at rest with considerably reduced exercise capacity but only mildly increased cardiac size. These patients often have

limited scarring but marked ischemic dysfunction in non-scarred parts of the ventricles and may be helped by revascularization. Others have moderate or severe cardiomegaly, reduced cardiac index, and elevation of right atrial pressure with hepatomegaly and fluid retention. Members of this latter group usually have extensive myocardial scarring

Table 2
Relationship between infarct size and mortality

	3-year mortality value (%)	P value
MI or scar >23%	43	.014
MI or scar <23%	5	
EF ≤43%	38	.029
EF >43%	6	
EF ≤43% without viable myocardium	63	.059
EF ≤43% with viable myocardium[a]	13	

Abbreviations: CABG, coronary artery bypass; EF, ejection fraction; MI, myocardial infarction.

[a] For all patients who had viable myocardium, the 3-year mortality rate was 8% (80% had CABG). For patients who had only fixed scar, >23% mortality rate was 50% (P = .018). Only 40% had CABG with no difference in morality with or without CABG.

Data from Yoshida F, Gould KL. Quantitative relation of myocardial infarct size and myocardial viability log position emission tomography to left ventricular rejection fraction and 3 years mortality with and without revascularization. J Am Coll Cardiol 1993;22:984–7.

and an LVESVI greater than 150 mL/m² and are unlikely to be improved by revascularization alone. The degree of left ventricular dysfunction has well-defined impact on survival.

Myocardial ischemia, left ventricular shape and volume, and mitral regurgitation are each surgical targets and the key to symptomatic relief in patients who have ischemic cardiomyopathy. Summarized by Buckberg [28] as the "three V's" (vessels, ventricle, and valve), combined ventricular restoration surgery (VSR), mitral repair, and CABG already provide outcomes equivalent or better than cardiac transplantation.

Left ventricular volume also has an important bearing on outcome after surgery for idiopathic dilated cardiomyopathy (IDCM). Ventricular restoration surgery and mitral repair can be combined in IDCM patients using the septal anterior ventricular exclusion (SAVE) procedure [29]. This operation is based on myocardial fibrosis and impaired myocardial contraction in IDCM not being uniform in distribution. Yanagida and coworkers [30] have shown a heterogeneity of wall motion abnormality in idiopathic dilated cardiomyopathy with a less contractile septum than posteroinferior wall. Experience with partial left ventriculectomy (Batista operation) also highlighted a greater degree of interstitial fibrosis in the septum compared with the lateral wall. Suma and colleagues confirmed left ventricular size to be a strong determinant for survival in IDCM and suggested that a reduction in ventricular size (in combination with mitral repair) may be advantageous for patients who have greatly enlarged hearts. One

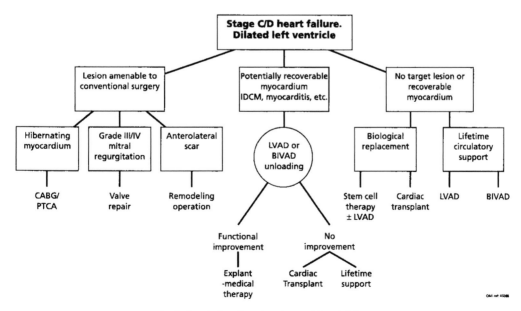

Fig. 7. Surgical options in advanced heart failure.

reason for failure of the Batista approach was that the most contractile part of the ventricle was excised during reduction of chamber size [31]. Accordingly Suma and colleagues [29] exclude akinetic septum by using a long narrow patch to provide a renewed ellipsoid shape.

The potential for myocardial recovery

For patients who have heart failure with IDCM, postpartum cardiomyopathy, viral myocarditis, or toxic cardiomyopathy, left or biventricular unloading with a circulatory assist device may improve or restore myocardial function [32]. Normalization of systemic blood flow gradually reverses multiorgan failure, improves coronary flow, and increases physical activity. Serum aldosterone, plasma rennin, atrial natriuretic peptide, and norepinephrine levels revert to normal as the heart failure syndrome disappears [4]. Until recently in the United States, transplantation was mandatory for all patients committed to an left ventricular assist device (LVAD). When the native heart was removed, it became clear to Frazier and others [33] that some ventricles with IDCM had reverted toward normal size and weight. Comparison of myocardial biopsies taken at LVAD implantation and during transplantation showed regression of myocyte hypertrophy, decreased myocytolysis, myocardial fibrosis, and apoptosis. Myocyte genetic expression and cellular metabolism reverted toward normal. Realization that recovering hearts were being discarded by transplantation led to the concept of mechanical bridge to myocardial recovery. Complimentary to this approach is the development of smaller more user-friendly axial flow and centrifugal blood pumps, which can be used for destination therapy if the myocardium fails to improve [6].

In IDCM patients, partial left ventricular unloading with a rotary blood pump achieves a symbiotic relationship between the native heart and the device. This approach has already provided event-free LVAD survival exceeding 6 years [34]. Most unloaded hearts show marginal improvement but some LVADs can be removed with prolonged survival. That an LVAD use does not preclude transplantation but paradoxically improves posttransplant survival opens the debate that circulatory support should be used primarily for IDCM patients, leaving transplantation in reserve [35].

Since the REMATCH trial, blood pumps are an accepted treatment for selected severely symptomatic non–transplant-eligible patients [36]. The prospects for bridge to recovery are critically dependent on myocardial pathology (Table 3). Patients in terminal decline with acute myocarditis or postpartum cardiomyopathy can be supported with an LVAD or biventricular assist device until resolution of the inflammatory process. These patients may have virtually normal left ventricular function after this salvage approach. Protocols to evaluate ventricular recovery have been developed by centers with active bridge to transplantation programs [37]. Patients who have an LVAD are initially followed with serial echocardiography, after which those who demonstrate signs of recovery are subject to more formal tests during exercise or dobutamine infusion. Candidates who have the potential for device explanation are fully heparinized (10,000 units intravenously) and the LVEF and left ventricular end diastolic dimension (LVEDD) are monitored while LVAD output is slowly decreased. If the patient remains stable on the lowest LVAD settings then support is discontinued for a period of 10 minutes to monitor unsupported left ventricular function. The weaning trial is halted if the LVEF falls below 40% or if the LVEDD increases greater than 55 mm. The trial suggests the potential for device explanation if the LVEF remains greater than 45% and the LVEDD less than 55 mm. LVAD support is then resumed for a longer period of device weaning while the left ventricle is subjected to an increasing amount of work before explanation.

Table 3
Potential for myocardial recovery in acute and chronic heart failure

	Recovery possible	Not recoverable
Acute heart failure	Acute myocarditis Myocardial infarction Postpartum CM Postcardiotomy shock	Giant cell myocarditis
Chronic heart failure	Idiopathic dilated CM Alcoholic CM	Ischemic CM Amyloidosis/ sarcoidosis Restrictive CM

Abbreviation: CM, cardiomyopathy.

In their weaning study, the Hetzer Group compared factors that distinguished those who had sustained recovery from others who reverted to heart failure [38]. Patients who remained well were younger, had a shorter history of heart failure, had a more rapid improvement in cardiac performance, and needed a shorter duration of LVAD support before indices of cardiac volume and function justified device removal. Duration over which the autoantibody against the β-adrenergic receptor disappeared from the serum was shorter (8.8 weeks versus 9.7 weeks) in patients who had sustainable recovery. Not different were mean age (41.5 years versus 50.3 years), mean LVEDD at the time of LVAD implantation (75.2 mm versus 78.7 mm), LVEF (14.8% versus 17.0%), and mean LVEDD 2 months after LVAD placement (53.7 mm versus 55.6 mm). They concluded that an LVAD unloading period of between 8 and 10 weeks was optimal for patients who had IDCM destined for sustainable recovery and that longer support could lead to myocyte atrophy.

Others have reservations about this limited duration and report success after much longer periods. Madegan and colleagues [39] studied explanted LVAD unloaded hearts between 8 to 155 days and found structural reverse remodeling to be complete in approximately 40 days. Both left ventricular chamber size and myocyte size had stabilized during this period. Collagen content was significantly increased in hearts supported for more than 40 days and this was consistent with a decrease in matrix metalloproteinase activity. Sarcoplasmic endoreticular calcium ATPase (SERCA2a) expression increased to normal levels by approximately 20 days of LVAD unloading. Although this information is difficult to translate into clinical practice, all patients who have idiopathic dilated cardiomyopathy who undergo LVAD implantation should be regarded as potential candidates for weaning without any certainty of reaching this goal.

Many serum markers have been shown to be pathologically elevated at the time of LVAD implantation and are improved or normalized by the time of removal [40]. These included TNFα, matrix metalloproteinases 2 and 9, metallothionein, beta receptor density and responsiveness, apoptosis, atrial natriuretic factor, nitric oxide synthase, IL-6, and annexins 1, 2, 4, and 6. None of these parameters are predictive in determining the reversibility of cardiac malfunction before LVAD implantation, however. Rather, they are markers of chronic LV overload and sympathetic nervous system hyperactivity. As such they may be useful to discriminate between patients who have reversed remodeling and those who remain dilated during mechanical unloading.

The Berlin Group considers the reversal of the inflammatory state in IDCM as essential for reverse remodeling. To achieve this they have treated IDCM patients with immunoadsorption to remove the autoantibodies. The treatment algorithm begins with optimal medical management. If this fails to improve cardiac status and pathologic levels of β1-autoantibodies are demonstrated, immunoadsorption is used. If cardiac function cannot be stabilized and cardiac transplantation criteria are met, the patient is placed on the waiting list and mechanical support is instituted with a hope of reversing the progressive cardiac impairment. The decision to insert an LVAD should not wait for terminal decline because the prospect for reversal of remodeling deteriorates with time. Aggressive medical and antioxidative treatment is pursued to enhance the chances of reverse remodeling.

Hetzer and colleagues reported successful explantation of 33 LVADs in patients who had dilated cardiomyopathy or myocarditis since 1995. The mean duration since device removal for all 33 patients was 6.5 years (range 1.3–9.3 years). Five-year survival after LVAD removal was 82%. Sustained improvement for more than 2 years after weaning occurred in 61% of the patients. The remainder relapsed into heart failure resulting in cardiac transplantation or death. When comparing patients who had long-term recovery versus those who relapsed, there were no differences regarding the mean age, mean LVEDD at the time of implantation, or mean LVEF. Many who relapsed already had severe myocardial fibrosis.

Although this pioneering work is promising, there are many further challenges. At present LVAD use is restricted to transplant centers and patients younger than 65 years. The vast majority of potential candidates miss the opportunity for this approach. Can the repair mechanism be enhanced to provide more predictable and sustained recovery? With newer more reliable LVADs should earlier LVAD unloading be used to improve the prospects for recovery? Can pharmacologic or stem cell treatment be used to promote recovery? Yacoub and colleagues have suggested the use of the anabolic β2-agonist clenbuterol to induce so-called "physiologic myocardial hypertrophy" during unloading [41]. In

rats the chronic administration of clenbuterol produces hypertrophy and increase SERCA2a content with a prolonged action potential and
increased oxidative carbohydrate use. In an un-
controlled study the Harefield Group combined
LVAD unloading and beta blockade followed by
clenbuterol administration to produce cardiac hypertrophy. With this regime the authors claim an
increased likelihood of sustainable myocardial recovery after LVAD removal. Despite this encouraging start, the overall prospect for recovery
remains limited as long as patients are left to absolute end stage before intervention [42].

Outcome after surgery for the three V's

The relationship between the extent of myocardial infarction, degree of left ventricular dysfunction, and late mortality was defined by
Yoshida and Gould [16]. They showed that a myocardial infarction of greater than 23% of the LV
circumference caused a decrease in LVEF (less
than 45%) and a 3-year mortality rate exceeding
40%. This finding contrasted with less extensive
myocardial infarctions, which carried a 3-year
mortality rate of only 5%. For patients in whom
LVEF was less than 43% the 3-year mortality
rate was 38% in contrast with only 6% when
LVEF was greater than 43%. LVEF alone was
a poor predictor of mortality in patients who
had hibernating myocardium. Viable myocardium
is an independent predictor of survival and
a marker for those who have impaired LVEF
who are most likely to benefit from revascularization. Three-year mortality rate in patients who
have LVEF of less than 43% and no viable myocardium is 63% in contrast to only 13% for those
who have viable myocardium submitted for revascularization. For patients who have only scar in
the territory at risk from coronary occlusion,
a 3-year mortality rate of 50% was no different
with or without revascularization, indicating no
benefit from CABG for this subgroup. These patients may nevertheless gain considerable improvement from left ventricular restoration
surgery to change a globular remodeled LV cavity
shape back to the more favorable elliptic configu-
ration. In this context Yamaguchi and colleagues
[43] in 1998 published 54% 5-year survival with
CABG alone for ischemic cardiomyopathy. Seven
years later the same authors reported 90% 5-year
survival for a similar patient group when left ventricular restoration and CABG were combined
[44].

In the presence of poor LV function without
angina or knowledge of regional myocardial
viability, it is unlikely that more than 50% of
patients will obtain benefit from CABG. Revascularization does not improve the function of scar
tissue and it is impossible by echocardiography,
coronary angiography, or ventriculography to
determine which areas of the myocardium might
benefit from improved perfusion. For patients
who had heart failure in the absence of limiting
angina, early studies suggested that CABG was
associated with poor short-term outcome and
a perioperative mortality rate of 15% to 20%
[27]. The goal of myocardial viability assessment
is to prospectively identify hibernating myocardium with the potential for functional improvement in patients whose prognosis may be
favorably altered by a high-risk operation. The
benefits of this approach were demonstrated by
Haas and colleagues [45] in a small series of 69
patients who had severe three-vessel disease and
LVEF less than 35%. Thirty-five patients were
operated on based on angiographic findings alone,
whereas 34 were selected by positron emission tomographic demonstration of hibernating myocardium and angiographic confirmation of favorable
target vessels. The hibernating myocardium group
had a lower hospital mortality rate (0% versus
11.4%, $P = .04$), a lower incidence of postoperative complications (33% versus 67%,
$P = .05$), and fewer patients who had low cardiac
output syndrome (3% versus 17%,
$P = .05$). Furthermore the 1-year survival rate
was better (97% ± 0.8% versus 79% ± 8%,
$P < .01$). The LVEF increased from 26% to
35% in those who had myocardial viability but
was unchanged in those who did not. This and
other supporting evidence indicate that assessment
of myocardial viability allows better definition of
risk and benefit of revascularization in patients
who have ischemic cardiomyopathy along with allowing refinement of patient selection in potential
transplant candidates. In turn functional magnetic
resonance imaging with assessment of left ventricular wall motion, thickness, and scar using gadolinium provides invaluable evidence of the potential
for wall motion improvement versus the need for
restoration surgery. Magnetic resonance imaging
also provides accurate assessment of the degree
and cause of mitral regurgitation.

Currently viability testing is indicated in those
heart failure patients who have suspected coronary disease or dilated cardiomyopathy who are
being considered for cardiac transplantation and

those who have known coronary disease and severe left ventricular dysfunction (LVEF less than 0.35) with breathlessness but only mild angina. Viability testing is redundant in patients who have unstable angina, postinfarction angina, or chronic stable angina, because revascularization is indicated for relief of symptoms. For ischemic patients who have heart failure symptoms but minimal angina, the combination of good target vessels with more than 25% myocardial viability suggests potential to benefit from CABG [46]. For those who have less than 25% viability or poor target vessels, or are reoperative candidates, surgery is unlikely to provide benefit.

Observational studies have documented substantial improvements in LV regional and global function following revascularization of hibernating myocardium [47,48]. This procedure provides relief from heart failure symptoms, improved survival, and important quality-of-life benefit. A comprehensive meta-analysis of largely retrospective data has been performed by Allman and colleagues [49]. In 24 studies reporting patient survival after viability testing, annual death rates were analyzed to produce a risk-adjusted relationship between the severity of LV dysfunction, presence of viability, and survival benefit associated with revascularization. The study included 3088 patients who had LVEF 32% ± 8% followed for 25 ± 10 months. For patients who had stunned or hibernating myocardium revascularization was associated with a 79.6% reduction in the annual mortality rate (16% versus 3.2%, $P < .0001$) compared with medical treatment. In contrast, patients who did not have viability had intermediate mortality, tending to higher rates with CABG versus medical therapy (7.7% versus 6.2%). Patients who had viability showed a direct relationship between the severity of LV dysfunction and magnitude of benefit with revascularization. No benefit was associated with revascularization in patients who did not have viability at any level of LVEF. The perioperative mortality rates were impressively high in patients who did not have viability (around 10%) but negligible in those who had viability. This difference in mortality is curious given the time frame of improvement in wall motion following revascularization.

Histopathologic studies have indicated a gradual increase in ultrastructural damage and degree of myocardial fibrosis as the ischemic process progresses through stunning, hibernation, nontransmural scar, and full-thickness scar [47].

Obviously scar never improves in function after revascularization even if covered with a veneer of healthy epicardial muscle following thrombolysis. Bax and colleagues [50] prospectively studied patients who had ischemic cardiomyopathy and left ventricular dysfunction using preoperative assessment of regional perfusion, glucose use, and contractile function. Of the dysfunctional segments, 22% were stunned, 23% were hibernating, and 55% were scar tissue. In stunned myocardium contractile function improved significantly at 3 months but without further improvement at 14 months. Some 30% of stunned segments did not improve. In hibernating segments 31% had improved by 3 months and 61% had recovered fully by 14 months. In a similar study using intraoperative myocardial biopsy from dysfunctional myocardium, Haas showed only 31% of stunned segments and 18% of hibernating segments to obtain complete functional recovery after 1 year [47]. Failure to improve was associated with more severe degenerative changes in the myocyte, including depletion of sarcomeres, accumulation of glycogen, loss of sarcoplasmic reticulum, and cellular sequestration. Using gadolinium-enhanced contrast MRI, Kim and colleagues [21] showed that 78% of dysfunctional segments identified as completely viable showed improvement in contractility after revascularization. In contrast, 90% of segments with 50% to 75% of wall thickness scar did not improve after revascularization.

The realization that the globular ischemic cardiomyopathy ventricle can be surgically restored to an elliptic shape by exclusion of scar is largely attributable to Dor [51]. Dor's endoventricular circular patch plasty followed pioneering attempts at physiologic reconstruction by Jatene and Cooley [52]. Dor's major contribution was to remove endocardial scar, exclude akinetic septum, restore the curvature of the anterolateral wall, and undertake complete myocardial revascularization and correction of mitral regurgitation. In the event of spontaneous or inducible ventricular tachycardia, cryotherapy was also applied to the edges of the resection (50% of cases). Between development of the surgical principles in 1984 and 2002, the Dor group operated on 1050 patients who were predominantly NYHA III or IV with LVEF less than 35%, LVESVI greater than 50 mL/m^2, LVEDVI greater than 100 mL/m^2, and mean pulmonary arterial pressure greater than 25 mm Hg [53]. One third of the cases had mitral regurgitation requiring repair. A balloon inflated to the theoretic diastolic capacity of the patient

(50 mL/m^2 body surface area) was used to avoid excessive reduction of chamber volume when rebuilding the ventricular cavity. By excluding akinetic or dyskinetic segments the procedure restored a more elliptic shape and improved contractile function. The mean improvement in LVEF in Dor's series was between 10% and 15%.

Surgical ventricular restoration (SVR) including coronary revascularization and mitral repair has been widely adopted as a mainstream heart failure procedure for ischemic cardiomyopathy. The RESTORE group registry contains more than 12,000 patients who had an overall 30-day mortality of 5% [54]. Mean LVESVI was reduced from 80 ± 51 mL/m^2 down to 57 ± 34 mL/m^2 providing an increase in LVEF of 29.6% ± 11.0% to 39% ± 12.3%. Five-year survival is 70%. Tulner and colleagues [55] have studied the acute changes in systolic and diastolic left ventricular mechanics using pressure volume loops before and after SVR. SVR provides acute volume reduction with shape alteration and decrease in ventricular dyssynchrony. All parameters of systolic function are improved but there is some increase in diastolic stiffness. SVR improved the mechanical efficiency of ventricular contraction although stroke work remained constant. This outcome contrasts with patients who undergo mitral annuloplasty alone in which only small changes in systolic function are observed [56]. Astrip and colleagues [57] used a mathematic model to study the differential effects of SVR on end-systolic and end-diastolic function. This model showed left ventricular mechanical synchrony to be substantially improved with marked beneficial effects for dyskinetic segments although less marked improvement for akinetic scar. When weak but contracting muscle was resected (as for the Batista operation), however, there was an overall negative effect on pump function.

For ischemic cardiomyopathy patients who have a dilated ventricle (LVESVI greater than 100 mL/m^2) SVR is clearly the most important component of the three V's. A recent study from O'Neill and colleagues [58] at the Cleveland Clinic emphasizes this fact. A total of 220 patients who had heart failure underwent SVR, of which 80% had concomitant CABG and 49% had mitral valve repair. Some 66% of these patients were NYHA III or IV, mean LVEF was 21.5% ± 7.3%, and mean LVEDD was 6.4 ± 1.0 cm. Thirty-day mortality was only 1% with 3- and 5-year survival of 90% and 80%, respectively. At follow-up 85% of patients were NYHA I or

II and postoperative left ventricular volume was the principal determinant of functional recovery during late follow-up. LVESVI was reduced from a mean value of 120 ± 46 mL/m^2 to 77 ± 26 mL/m^2 although the increase in LVEF was modest: 21.5% to 24.7% ($P < .01$). The authors concluded that these outcomes were better than those attained by committal to the transplant waiting list. The results are also substantially better than those presented by Gillinov and colleagues [59] for CABG and mitral valve repair in ischemic cardiomyopathy, in which 5-year survival was only 55%.

Ventricular volume is an important denominator of outcome after mitral repair for ischemic cardiomyopathy and IDCM [60]. Horii and colleagues [61] examined the relationship between LVESVI and functional recovery in 55 patients who had IDCM undergoing mitral repair or replacement, 38 of whom also required tricuspid valve surgery. These patients had a mean age of 55 years and were NYHA III or IV. Half were already on inotropic support. Preoperative LVESVI ranged from 70 to 270 mL/m^2. They were arbitrarily divided into two groups with LVESVI greater than or less than 150 mL/m^2. The small ventricle group had mean LVESVI of 114 ± 26 mL/m^2, whereas the large ventricle group had LVESVI 183 ± 36 mL/m^2. Hospital mortality was 4.3% for elective surgery and 14.5% for those on inotropes. For those who had LVESVI less than 150 mL/m^2 there was an improvement in LVEF from 24.6% to 30.4% and a concomitant fall in LVESVI from a mean of 114 mL/m^2 to 99 mL/m^2 at 1 year. In contrast the large LV group with LVESVI greater than 150 mL/m^2 or LVEDD greater than 70 mm had no significant benefit from mitral repair. This finding partially explains the variable results of mitral repair alone in other IDCM series.

Suma developed septal anterior ventricular exclusion (SAVE procedure) in an attempt to improve the outlook for Japanese patients who do not have access to cardiac transplantation [29]. The operation was applied to 36 NYHA III/IV patients (mean age 60 years) who had greater than 2+ mitral regurgitation. All had LVEDD greater than 77 mm and an akinetic septum. All patients had the SAVE procedure, 26 with mitral repair and 10 with mitral replacement. Sixteen also had tricuspid repair. Operative mortality was 13.8% but 60% of those needing urgent surgery died. Nevertheless 1- and 3-year survival rates were 67.5% and 60.7%, respectively, and survivors were NYHA I or II. There was a marked improvement in left ventricular volume and function. LVEF improved from 20.9% ± 6.4% to 27.5% ± 8.8%, whereas LVEDP fell from 24.3 ± 9.7 mm Hg to 19.4 ± 7.6 mm Hg. Mean LVESVI was reduced from 181.3 ± 55.4 mL/m^2 to 133 ± 54.1 mL/m^2. There was no significant redilation of the ventricle at 3 years. Once again postoperative left ventricular volume was the strongest determinant for late survival. This survival was 67% in those who had LVESVI less than 150 mL/m^2 and only 42% for those who had LVESVI greater than 150 mL/m^2. It is possible that IDCM patients who had larger ventricles would be better candidates for long-term circulatory support with a rotary blood pump.

The question as to whether external ventricular constraint could add additional benefit to mitral repair has been addressed in the Acorn clinical trial [62]. This was a randomized study of NYHA III/IV patients who had LVEF less than 35% (mean 23% ± 9%) who received mitral repair with or without the restraining Acorn polyester mesh. In short, external restraint provided no additional benefit greater than mitral repair alone.

What can be done for those who do not have a target lesion or recoverable myocardium?

Currently there are two established options: cardiac transplantation or lifetime mechanical circulatory support [63,64]. A third possibility is that of cellular therapy and myocardial tissue engineering [65]. This option may be supported by mechanical left ventricular unloading to reduce LVEDP and promote myocardial blood flow in an attempt to sustain the transplanted cells.

Cardiac transplantation is covered in detail in elsewhere in this issue. A donor heart provides symptomatic relief with contemporary survival exceeding 80% at 1 year and almost 50% at 10 years [63]. The operation is largely restricted to patients less than 65 years of age. By the very nature of heart failure, 80% of patients are older than 65 years and younger patients often have comorbidities, such as renal impairment or diabetes, which preclude them from transplantation [66]. Given the developments in SVR, the evidence base for transplantation is less secure than it was 30 years ago. Clear indications include refractory cardiogenic shock, dependence on intravenous inotropic support (both Status I) or persistent Class IV symptoms with a peak oxygen consumption of

less than 10 mL/kg/min [67]. Without treatment these patients have a projected outcome that varies from imminent death to greater than 50% mortality at 6 months. In contrast, most candidates have been ambulatory on oral medical therapy (Status II) and have less impaired peak oxygen consumption (11–14 mL/kg/min). For these patients the benefits of a transplant waiting list are less apparent, particularly if they have a target lesion or potentially recoverable myocardium (IDCM or myocarditis). Deng and colleagues [68] showed that Status II German patients who were on a waiting list but did not receive an organ had a similar 3- and 4-year risk-adjusted survival rate to those who were transplanted. As many as 30% of Status II patients improved symptomatically and prognostically when provided with the medical management of an expert heart failure team at a transplant unit. Patients are deemed too well for transplantation if they show a sustained improvement of peak oxygen uptake of greater than 2 mL/kg/min. Shah and colleagues [69] showed that 1- and 3-year survival for Status II patients removed from the waiting list was 100% and 92%, respectively. Those who had IDCM frequently showed spontaneous improvement with much better long-term outlook than for ischemic cardiomyopathy.

The prospects for lifetime mechanical circulatory support are continuously improving [70]. Blood pump bioengineering has developed rapidly in recent years and there are many new LVADs undergoing bench, animal, or clinical testing. Much smaller continuous flow devices have been developed with blood-washed micro-ceramic bearings, electromagnetic suspension, and now hydrodynamic suspension to provide durability and minimal thrombogenicity [6]. The power packs and controllers are easily portable. The risk for power-line infection has been reduced by finer, more flexible electric cables, transcutaneous energy transmission, or skull-mounted pedestals. As an off-the-shelf commodity, LVAD use could exceed transplantation by a factor of 50 to 1. Although survival benefit was clearly shown in the REMATCH study, quality of life was limited by LVAD-related complications [36]. Chronic infection caused 41% of LVAD deaths and by two years the probability of LVAD mechanical failure was 35%. There was a 42% incidence of bleeding complications by 6 months and an overall stroke rate of 10%. Many of these problems were inherent in the design and power supply of the first generation pulsatile blood pump designed in the 1980s. During the course of REMATCH recruitment it was clear that early mortality occurred largely through failure to resurrect moribund patients who had multiorgan failure [71]. With more sensible patient selection an initial 2-year survival of 21% improved to 43% late in the recruitment phase. By implanting before terminal decline and with improved postoperative management, the University of Utah achieves 85% 1-year and 65% 2-year survival with the same device.

Refinement of LVAD technology has already improved outcomes. The first patient to receive a permanent Jarvik Flowmaker in the United Kingdom remains active in the community after almost 7 years of event-free survival [34]. Skull pedestal power delivery allows all external components (power line, batteries, and controller) to be exchanged, an important option in lifetime support. Other rotary blood pumps, including Thermocardio Systems II, Berlin Incor, Ventracor, and Terumo LVADs, are in clinical use for bridge to transplantation or lifetime support [6]. Concern that pulse pressure is required to maintain end organ function in the human have been dispelled by laboratory and clinical experience [72]. Mechanical reliability and resistance to infection are impressive. In the first 150 Jarvik Flowmaker patients there has been no blood pump malfunction. The remaining issue of thromboembolism is being addressed by device modifications and improved anticoagulant regimes. These noiseless, easily portable, and user-friendly rotary blood pumps allow the patient to live an unrestricted and productive life, including long-haul air travel.

Analysis of mortality in LVAD patients shows that many die from irreversible organ dysfunction already present at the time of device implantation [36]. Patients considered for lifetime LVAD use have by protocol been ineligible for cardiac transplantation and in an advanced state of decompensation. Many have multisite pacing, an implantable defibrillator, or are confined to hospital with intravenous inotropes or an intra-aortic balloon pump. As such they have been left too late. The REMATCH study suggested that when a patient is considered unsuitable for transplantation by the same argument they may also have an unreasonably high risk for LVAD surgery [36]. The decision to proceed to lifetime circulatory support should be made on an elective basis, not as a salvage procedure [73]. With safer more user-friendly devices and less invasive operations, LVAD deployment should be brought forward

out of the end-stage arena [35]. Given that circulatory support and rehabilitation have improved the results of cardiac transplantation it is illogical and perhaps unethical to exclude transplant-eligible patients from clinical trials of LVAD therapy. Some LVAD patients inevitably require transplantation because of progressive right heart failure. Other individuals who have been excluded from transplantation through renal impairment or increased pulmonary vascular resistance can improve sufficiently to attain transplant status.

Preliminary evidence suggests that LVADs are cost effective by reducing hospital admissions and in some cases returning young patients to employment [34]. Multisite pacing and implantable defibrillators are already widely accepted despite their limited symptomatic benefit [74]. Blood pumps provide better symptomatic relief and further clinical trials are needed to determine the survival benefit conferred by safer devices. The future lies with yet smaller pumps, which can be implanted without major surgery in these high-risk patients. Although the economic implications of widespread LVAD use are substantial, other treatments for terminal illness already set the precedent. Hemodialysis is extensively used for maintenance treatment of renal failure patients irrespective of age, providing 60% 2-year survival [75].

Myocardial regeneration: future potential

Cardiac regeneration using cell therapy to replace lost myocardial mass has the potential to revolutionize the treatment of heart failure [76]. Cellular cardiomyoplasty has moved from bench to bedside extremely rapidly, generating more questions than answers [77]. Clinical studies have shown small but consistent improvements in mechanical function, largely independent of the cell type chosen [78–80]. Choosing the best cell type for repair may depend on the nature of injury. In conditions in which chronic ischemia prevails and angiogenesis is a partial objective, the angiogenic potential of nonmyogenic bone marrow–derived cells is promising [81]. In these circumstances bone marrow mononuclear cells, endothelial or vascular progenitor cells from bone marrow or blood, marrow angioblasts, or blood-derived multipotent adult progenitor cells may prove optimal [82]. For most patients an improvement in contractile function is the primary goal [83]. Skeletal myoblasts have been used clinically but do not make connexins, the building blocks of gap junctions, and are therefore unlikely to make electrical connections with the native myocardium [84]. Although several reports have documented improved mechanical function with these cells, improvement is likely to be the result of a passive mechanism and not because of contractile mass [85]. Other contractile options include cardiac stem cells and other mesenchymal progenitors, which may develop down the myogenic line [86–88].

To produce mechanical work, the cell must be excited in synchrony with the native myocardium, and this requires integration by way of gap junctions [84]. The cells must also have longitudinal shortening capability through development of sarcomeres. They must be aligned with appropriate geometry to provide contractile function and achieve integration without the dysrhythmic potential inherent in skeletal myoblasts. Cardiac stem cells, mesenchymal stem cells, and embryonic stem cells each have the potential to provide exogenous contractile mass to integrate within the myocardium [80,82,87]. Mesenchymal and hematopoietic stem cells also contribute to angiogenesis and may produce paracrine factors that promote native cell survival. No new myocytes are produced and angiogenesis alone cannot restore contractile myocardium [89,90].

One of the principle problems with cell transplantation is poor survival of the new cells. Most reports suggest that 70% to 90% of transplanted cells die within the first few days after introduction into the infarct scar [91,92]. Injected cells are exposed to an ischemic environment with elevated wall tension [93]. The more undifferentiated and ischemia-resistant a cell is, the higher its engraftment rate. The more differentiated a cell is toward a cardiac phenotype the lower is its resistance, and engraftment is poor. An ideal cell would be ischemia resistant initially and become fully functional after engraftment. Alternatively, combinations of cells could be used to modify the local environment, providing angiogenesis and myoblast contractile potential.

Multiple attempts have already been made to increase the angiogenic potential of skeletal myoblasts by inducing the expression of the pro-angiogenic molecule, vascular endothelial growth factor. Combinations of angiogenic bone marrow and myogenic muscle–derived cells are promising. Bonaros and colleagues combined transplantation of homologous skeletal myoblasts with human AC-133+ cells in experimental myocardial infarction [94]. The combination of skeletal myoblasts and angiopoietic progenitor cells resulted in improvement in ventricular function, reduction in scar size, increased neo-angiogenesis, and decreased rates of apoptosis in the engrafted myotubes. The authors attributed functional improvement to the improved blood supply for the engrafted myoblasts in the scar tissue. In the same volume of the *Journal of Thoracic and Cardiovascular Surgery*, Huang and colleagues [95] described a synergistic effect between transplanted autologous mesenchymal stem cells transfected with the angiogenin gene in comparison with the stem cell injection alone. In a pig myocardial infarction model both groups experienced decreased scar size, increased scar thickness, and improved cardiac function, but the synergistic effect of stem cells with angiogenin was manifest by increased myocardial perfusion and significantly better left ventricular mechanics. Transplantation of the mesenchymal stem cells overexpressing angiogenin clearly produced stronger beneficial effects on ventricular modulation and myocardial reperfusion. The novel combination of cell therapy with gene transfection is a promising strategy to restore cardiac function in chronic myocardial ischemia and may prove even more effective in an unloaded ventricle.

Given the enormous potential for cell therapy and the progress made with circulatory support devices, it is possible that the surgical treatment of heart failure may change dramatically in the next decade. For cell therapy to reach its potential, selection of cell type maximizing survival and promoting differentiation of progenitor cells down cardiomyocyte or cardiovascular cell pathways is necessary. Electrical integration and coordination with native myocardium remains a substantial challenge. There are several potential delivery options for cells and genes and if left ventricular unloading can improve cell survival the whole field should remain in the surgical arena. Cell culture techniques and tissue bioengineering may ultimately produce sheets of contracting myocytes that can be grafted surgically into the failing heart [96].

In summary modern imaging has highlighted the relationship between left ventricular shape, volume, and prognosis. Substantial clinical research supported by computer modeling has defined the benefits of VRS in ischemic and idiopathic dilated cardiomyopathies. Of the three V's—vessel, valve and ventricle—reduction in left ventricular volume seems to convey most prognostic benefit. Although most surgeons have expertise in CABG and mitral repair there seems to be considerably less understanding of volume-reduction surgery, particularly for IDCM. For the future the combination of mechanical left ventricular unloading (with yet unforeseen LVADs), together with myocardial tissue engineering, holds great promise.

In the meantime cardiac transplantation provides the benchmark for heart failure survival but donor availability has not increased despite the use of older donors. The 2000 carefully selected recipients each year in the United States have an 87% probability of surviving the first year, a half-life in excess of 10 years, and a high probability of an excellent quality of life. In the words of Sharon Hunt from the *New England Journal of Medicine*, "for younger patients without serious coexisting conditions who are willing to submit to the requirement of a lifetime of medication and medical care, this possibility is an outstanding alternative to early death" [63].

References

[1] Bailey CP, Gilman RA. Experimental and clinical resection for ventricular aneurysm. Surg Gynecol Obstet 1957;104:539–42.

[2] Westaby S. The foundations of cardiac surgery. Landmarks of cardiac surgery. Oxford (UK): Isis Medical Media Ltd; 1997. p. 1–48.

[3] Stewart S. Financial aspects of heart failure programs of care. Eur J Heart Fail 2005;7:423–8.

[4] Muller J, Wallukat G, Weng Y, et al. Weaning from mechanical cardiac support in patients with idiopathic dilated cardiomyopathy. Circulation 1997; 96:542–9.

[5] Athanasuleas CL, Buckberg GD, Menicanti L, et al. Optimising ventricular shape in anterior restoration. Semin Thorac Cardiovasc Surg 2001;13(4):459–67.

[6] Westaby S. Ventricular assist device as destination therapy. Surg Clin North Am 2004;84:91–123.

[7] ACC/AHA. Guidelines for the evaluation and management of chronic heart failure in adults: executive summary. J Am Cardiol 2001;38:2101–13.

[8] The SEOSI Investigators. Survey on heart failure in Italian hospital cardiology units. Eur Heart J 1997; 18:1457–64.

[9] Senni M, Redfield MM. Heart failure with preserved systolic function: a different natural history? J Am Coll Cardiol 2001;38:1277–82.

[10] Owan TE, Hodge DO, Hergos RM, et al. Trends in prevalence and outcome of heart failure with preserved ejection fraction. N Engl J Med 2006;355: 251–9.

[11] Bhatia RS, Vu JV, Lee DS, et al. Outcome of heart failure with preserved ejection fraction in a population based study. N Engl J Med 2006;355:260–9.

[12] Katz AM. Pathophysiology of heart failure: identifying targets for pharmacotherapy. Med Clin North Am 2003;87:303–16.

[13] Gerdes AM, Capasso JM. Structural remodelling and mechanical dysfunction of cardiac myocytes in heart failure. J Mol Cell Cardiol 1995;27:849–56.

[14] Bolling SF, Pagani FD', Deeb GM, et al. Intermediate term outcome of mitral reconstruction in cardiomyopathy. J Thorac Cardiovasc Surg 1998;111: 381–8.

[15] Dec GW, Fuster Y. Idiopathic dilated cardiomyopathy. N Engl J Med 1994;331:1564–75.

[16] Yoshida F, Gould KL. Quantitative relation of myocardial infarct size and myocardial viability by positron emission tomography to left ventricular ejection fraction and 3 year mortality with and without revascularization. J Am Coll Cardiol 1993;22: 984–97.

[17] Walker CA, Crawford FA, Spinale FG. Myocyte contractile dysfunction with hypertrophy and failure: relevance to cardiac surgery. J Thorac Cardiovasc Surg 2000;119:388–400.

[18] White HD, Norris RM, Brown MA, et al. Left ventricular and systolic volume as the major determinant of survival after recovery from myocardial infarction. Circulation 1987;76:44–51.

[19] Edmond M, Mock MB, Davis KB, et al. Long-term survival of medically treated patients in the coronary artery surgery study (CASS). Circulation 1994;90: 2645–57.

[20] Bonow RO. Myocardial viability and prognosis in patients with ischemic left ventricular dysfunction. J Am Coll Cardiol 2002;39:1159–62.

[21] Kim RJ, Wu E, Rafael A, et al. The use of contrast-enhanced magnetic resonance imaging to identify reversible myocardial dysfunction. N Engl J Med 2000;343:1445–53.

[22] Hausmann H, Topp H, Siniaswski H, et al. Decision making in end stage coronary artery disease. revascularisation or heart transplantation. Ann Thorac Surg 1997;64:1296–302.

[23] Franciosa JA, Wilen M, Ziesche S, et al. Survival in men with severe chronic left ventricular failure due to either coronary heart disease or idiopathic dilated cardiomyopathy. Am J Cardiol 1983;51:831–6.

[24] Garg R, Yusuf S. Overview of randomized trials on angiotensin-converting enzyme inhibitors on mortality and morbidity in patients with heart failure. JAMA 1995;273:1450–6.

[25] CIBIS-II investigators and committees. The cardiac insufficiency bisoprolol study II (CIBIS-II): a randomised trial. Lancet 1999;353:9–13.

[26] Packer M, Carver R, Rodeheffer J, et al. Effect of oral milrinone on mortality in severe chronic heart failure. The PROMISE study research group. N Engl J Med 1991;325:1450–6.

[27] Westaby S. Coronary revascularization in ischemic cardiomyopathy. Surg Clin North Am 2004;84:179–99.

[28] Buckberg G. Left ventricular reconstruction for dilated ischaemic cardiomyopathy: biology, registry, randomisation and credibility. Eur J Thorac Cardiovasc Surg 2006;30:753–61.

[29] Suma H, Isomura T, Horii T, et al. Septal anterior ventricular exclusion procedure for idiopathic dilated cardiomyopathy. Ann Thorac Surg 2006;82:1344–8.

[30] Yanagida R, Sugawara M, Kawai A, et al. Regional differences in myocardial work of the left ventricle in patients with idiopathic dilated cardiomyopathy: implications for the surgical technique used for left ventriculoplasty. J Thorac Cardiovasc Surg 2001;122:600–7.

[31] Gorcsan J, Feldman AM, Kormos RL, et al. Heterogeneous immediate effects of partial left ventriculectomy on cardiac performance. Circulation 1998;97:839–42.

[32] Bartling B, Milting H, Schumann H, et al. Myocardial gene expression of regulators of myocyte apoptosis and myocyte calcium homeostasis during hemodynamic unloading by left ventricular assist devices in patients with end stage heart failure. Circulation 1999;100:216–23.

[33] Frazier OH, Benedict CR, Radovancevic B, et al. Improved left ventricular function after chronic left ventricular unloading. Ann Thorac Surg 1996;62:675–82.

[34] Westaby S, Frazier OH, Banning A. Six years of continuous circulatory support. N Engl J Med 2006;355:325–7.

[35] Frazier OH, Rose EH, MCCarthy PM, et al. Improved mortality and rehabilitation of transplant candidates treated with long term implantable left ventricular assist system. Ann Thorac Surg 1995;222:327–38.

[36] Rose EA, Gelijns AC, Moskowitz AJ, et al. Randomized evaluation of mechanical assistance for the treatment of congestive heart failure (REMATCH) study group. Long-term mechanical left ventricular assistance for end-stage heart failure. N Engl J Med 2001;345:1435–43.

[37] Hetzer R, Muller J, Weng Y, et al. Cardiac recovery in dilated cardiomyopathy by unloading with a left ventricular assist device. Ann Thorac Surg 1999;68:742–9.

[38] Loebe M, Muller J, Hetzer R. Ventricular assistance for recovery of cardiac failure. Curr Opin Cardiol 1999;14:234–48.

[39] Madegan JD, Barbone A, Choudhri AF, et al. Time course of reverse remodelling of the left ventricle during support with a left ventricular assist device. J Thorac Cardiovasc Surg 2001;121:902–8.

[40] Zhang J, Narula J. Molecular biology of myocardial recovery. Surg Clin North Am 2004;84:223–42.

[41] Birks EJ, Tansley PD, Hardy J, et al. Left ventricular assist device and drug therapy for the reversal of heart failure. N Engl J Med 2006;355:1873–84.

[42] Mancini DM, Beniaminovitz A, Levin H, et al. Low incidence of myocardial recovery after left ventricular assist device implantation in patients with chronic heart failure. Circulation 1998;98:2383–9.

[43] Yamaguchi A, Ino T, Adachi H, et al. Left ventricular volume predicts postoperative course in patients with ischaemic cardiomyopathy. Ann Thorac Surg 1998;65:434–8.

[44] Yamaguchi A, Adachi H, Kawahito K, et al. Left ventricular reconstruction benefits patients with dilated ischaemic cardiomyopathy. Ann Thorac Surg 2005;79(2):456–61.

[45] Haas F, Haetinel CJ, Picker W, et al. Preoperative positron emission tomographic viability assessment and perioperative risk in patients with advanced ischemic heart disease. J Am Coll Cardiol 1997;30:1693–700.

[46] Lee KS, Marwick TH, Cook SA, et al. Prognosis of patients with left ventricular dysfunction, with and without viable myocardium after myocardial infarction. Relative efficacy of medical therapy and revascularisation. Circulation 1994;90:2687–94.

[47] Haas F, Jennen L, Heinzmann U, et al. Ischemically compromised myocardium displays different time-courses of functional recovery: correlation with morphological alterations? Eur J Cardiothorac Surg 2001;20:290–8.

[48] Arnese M, Cornel JH, Salustri A, et al. Prediction of improvement of regional left ventricular function after surgical revascularisation. A comparison of low-dose dobutamine echocardiography with 201T1 single-photon emission computed tomography. Circulation 1995;91:2748–52.

[49] Allman KC, Shaw LJ, Hachamovitch R, et al. Myocardial viability testing and impact of revascularisation on prognosis in patients with coronary artery disease and left ventricular dysfunction: a meta-analysis. J Am Coll Cardiol 2002;39:1151–8.

[50] Bax JJ, Visser FC, Poldermans D, et al. Time course of functional recovery of stunned and hibernating segments after surgical revascularisation. Circulation 2001;104(Suppl 1):314–8.

[51] Dor V, Saab M, Coste P, et al. Left ventricular aneurysm: a new surgical approach. Thorac Cardiovasc Surg 1989;37:11–9.

[52] Jatene AD. Left ventricular aneurysmectomy: resection or reconstruction. J Thorac Cardiovasc Surg 1985;89:321–31.

[53] Dor V. Surgical remodeling of the left ventricle. Surg Clin North Am 2004;84:27–43.

[54] Athanasuleas CL, Stanley AW Jr, Buckberg GD, et al. Surgical anterior ventricular endocardial restoration (SAVER) in the dilated remodeled ventricle after anterior myocardial infarction. RESTORE group. Reconstructive ENDOVENTRICULAR surgery, returning torsion original radius elliptical shape to the LV. J Am Coll Cardiol 2001;36:2098–103.

[55] Tulner SA, Steendijk P, Klautz RJ, et al. Surgical ventricular restoration in patients with ischemic dilated cardiomyopathy: evaluation of systolic and diastolic ventricular function, wall stress, dyssynchrony, and mechanical efficiency by

pressure-volume loops. J Thorac Cardiovasc Surg 2006;132(3):610–20.

[56] Bach DS, Bolling SF. Early improvement in congestive heart failure after correction of secondary mitral regurgitation in end stage cardiomyopathy. Am Heart J 1995;129:1165–70.

[57] Astrip JH, Oz M, Burkhoff D. Left ventricular volume reduction surgery for heart failure: a physiologic perspective. J Thorac Cardiovasc Surg 2001;122: 775–82.

[58] O'Neill JO, Starling RC, McCarthy PM, et al. The impact of left ventricular reconstruction on survival in patients with ischemic cardiomyopathy. Eur J Cardiothorac Surg 2006;30:753–61.

[59] Gillinov AM, Faber C, Houghtaling PL, et al. Repair versus replacement for degenerative mitral valve disease with coexisting ischemic heart disease. J Thorac Cardiovasc Surg 2003;125(6): 1350–62.

[60] Braun J, Bax JJ, Versteegh MIM, et al. Preoperative left ventricular dimensions predict reverse remodelling following restrictive mitral annuloplasty in ischaemic mitral regurgitation. Eur J Cardiothorac Surg 2005;27:847–58.

[61] Horii T, Suma H, Isomura T, et al. Left ventricular volume affects the result of mitral valve surgery for idiopathic dilated cardiomyopathy to treat congestive heart failure. Ann Thorac Surg 2006;82: 1349–55.

[62] Grossi EA, Crooke GA. Mitral valve surgery in heart failure: insights from the ACORN clinical trial. J Thorac Cardiovasc Surg 2006;132:455–6.

[63] Hunt SA. Taking heart—cardiac transplantation, past, present and future. N Engl J Med 2006;355: 231–5.

[64] Deng MC, Young JB, Stevenson LW, et al. Board of directors of the international society for heart and lung transplantation destination mechanical circulatory support: proposal for clinical standards. J Heart Lung Transplant 2003;22:365–9.

[65] Wu KH, Liu YL, Zhou B, et al. Cellular therapy and myocardial tissue engineering: the role of adult stem and progenitor cells. Eur J Cardiothorac Surg 2006; 30:770–81.

[66] Redfield MM. Heart failure—an epidemic of uncertain proportions. N Engl J Med 2002;347:1442–4.

[67] Miller LW. Patient selection for the use of ventricular assist devices as a bridge to transplantation. Ann Thorac Surg 2003;75:S66–71.

[68] Deng MC, De Meester JMJ, Smits JMA, et al. For the COCPIT study group. The effect of receiving a heart transplant: analysis of a cohort entered onto a waiting list, stratified by heart failure severity. BMJ 2000;321:540–5.

[69] Shah NR, Rogers JD, Eward GA, et al. Survival of patients removed from the heart transplant waiting list. J Thorac Cardiovasc Surg 2004;127: 1481–5.

[70] Lietz K, Miller LW. Will left ventricular assist device therapy replace heart transplantation in the foreseeable future? Curr Opin Cardiol 2005;20:132–7.

[71] Stevenson LW, Miller LW, Desvigne-Nickens P, et al. Left ventricular assist device as destination for patients undergoing intravenous inotropic therapy: a subset analysis from REMATCH (Randomised Evaluation of Mechanical Assistance in Treatment of Chronic Heart Failure). Circulation 2004;110:975–81.

[72] Saito S, Nishinkaka T, Westaby S. Hemodynamics of chronic non-pulsatile blood flow: implications for LVAD development. Surg Clin North Am 2004;84:61–74.

[73] Jurmann MJ, Weng Y, Drews T, et al. Permanent mechanical circulatory support in patients of advanced age. Eur J Cardiothorac Surg 2004;25:610–8.

[74] Greenberg B, Mehra MR. All patients with heart failure and intraventricular conduction defect or dyssynchrony should not receive cardiac resynchronisation therapy. Circulation 2006;114:2685–91.

[75] The United States Renal Data System. 2004 Annual data report. Available at: http://www.usrds.org/. Accessed June 1, 2007.

[76] Siminiak S, Kurpisz M. Myocardial replacement therapy. Circulation 2003;108:1167–71.

[77] Hagege AA, Marolleau JP, Vilquin JT, et al. Skeletal myoblast transplantation in ischaemic heart failure: long term follow up of the first phase I cohort of patients. Circulation 2006;114(Suppl 1):108–13.

[78] Menasche P, Hagege AA, Vilquin JT, et al. Autologous skeletal myoblast transplantation for severe postinfarction left ventricular dysfunction. J Am Coll Cardiol 2003;41:1078–83.

[79] Strauer BE, Brehm M, Zeus T, et al. Repair of infarcted myocardium by autologous intracoronary mononuclear bone marrow cell transplantation in humans. Circulation 2002;106:1913–8.

[80] Thompson RB, Emani SM, Davis BH, et al. Comparison of intracardiac cell transplantation: autologous skeletal myoblasts versus bone marrow cells. Circulation 2003;108(Suppl 1):11264–71.

[81] Kocher AA, Schuster MD, Szabolcs MJ, et al. Neovascularisation of ischaemic myocardium by human bone-marrow-derived angioblasts prevents cardiomyocyte apoptosis, reduces remodelling and improves cardiac function. Nat Med 2001;7:430–6.

[82] Beltrami AP, Barlucchi L, Torella D, et al. Adult cardiac stem cells are multipotent and support myocardial regeneration. Cell 2003;114:763–76.

[83] Anversa P, Nadal-Ginard B. Myocyte renewal and ventricular remodeling. Nature 2002;415:240–3.

[84] Valiunas V, Doronin S, Valiuniene L, et al. Human mesenchymal stem cells make cardiac connexins and form functional gap junctions. J Physiol 2004;555: 617–26.

[85] Gaudette GR, Cohen IS. Cardiac regeneration: materials can improve the passive properties of

myocardium but cell therapy must do more. Circulation 2006;114:2575–7.

[86] Anversa P, Kajstura J, Leri A, et al. Life and death of cardiac stem cells: a paradigm shift in cardiac biology. Circulation 2006;113:1451–63.

[87] Silva GV, Litovsky S, Assad JA, et al. Mesenchymal stem cells differentiate into an endothelial phenotype, enhance vascular density, and improve heart function in a canine chronic ischemia model. Circulation 2005;11:150–6.

[88] Woller KC, Drexler H. Clinical applications of stem cells for the heart. Circ Res 2005;96:151–63.

[89] Murray CE, Soonpaa MH, Reinecke H, et al. Haematopoietic stem cells do not transdifferentiate into cardiac myocytes in myocardial infarcts. Nature 2004;428:664–8.

[90] Deten A, Volz HC, Clamors S, et al. Hematopoietic stem cells do not repair the infarcted mouse heart. Cardiovasc Res 2005;65:52–63.

[91] Agbulut O, Vandervelde S, Al Attar N, et al. Comparison of human skeletal myoblasts and bone marrow derived CD133+ progenitors for the repair of infarcted myocardium. J Am Coll Cardiol 2004;44: 458–63.

[92] Fernandez-Aviles F, San Roman JA, Garcia-Frade J, et al. Experimental and clinical regenerative capability of human bone marrow cells after myocardial infarction. Circ Res 2004;95:742–8.

[93] Wollert KC, Meyer GP, Lotz J, et al. Intracoronary autologous bone marrow cell transfer after myocardial infarction: the BOOST randomised controlled clinical trial. Lancet 2004;364:141–8.

[94] Bonaros N, Rauf D, Wolf E, et al. Combined transplantation of skeletal myoblasts and angiopoietic progenitor cells reduces infarct size and apoptosis and improves cardiac function in chronic ischaemic heart failure. J Thorac Cardiovasc Surg 2006;132: 1321–8.

[95] Huang SD, Lu FL, Xu X, et al. Transplantation of angiogenin-overexpressing mesenchymal stem cells synergistically augments cardiac function in a porcine model of chronic ischaemia. J Thorac Cardiovasc Surg 2006;132:1329–47.

[96] Hata H, Matsumiya G, Miyagawa S, et al. Grafted skeletal myoblast sheets attenuate myocardial remodelling in pacing-induced canine heart failure model. J Thorac Cardiovasc Surg 2006; 132:918–24.

ELSEVIER
SAUNDERS

Heart Failure Clin 3 (2007) 159–180

HEART
FAILURE
CLINICS

Maximizing Survival Potential in Very High Risk Cardiac Surgery

Stephen Westaby, MS, PhD, FRCS*,
L. Balacumaraswami, MBBS, FRCS (C-Th), R. Sayeed, PhD, FRCS

Oxford Heart Centre, John Radcliffe Hospital, Oxford, UK

The mean age and risk profile of patients referred for cardiac surgery is constantly increasing. Surgeons are now inclined to accept high-risk patients because interventional cardiology provides less invasive alternatives for an overlapping patient cohort. As risk profile increases so does hospital mortality. A survey of 8641 patients who underwent coronary artery bypass operations in New England showed an overall mortality of 4.48%, of which 65% could be directly attributed to postcardiotomy myocardial failure [1]. In the PURSUIT trial, which randomized patients who had coronary bypass and unstable angina to a glycoprotein IIb/IIIa inhibitor or placebo, the 7-day mortality or myocardial infarction rate was 22.3% in almost 700 patients in the control arm [2]. A collective review of 279 patients who had dialysis-dependent coronary bypass reported a 12.2% hospital mortality [3]. Similarly the Mayo Clinic Group reported a 14% perioperative mortality for patients who had aortic valve replacement with a left ventricular ejection fraction (LVEF) less than 35% and a borderline transvalvular gradient [4]. Intraoperative myocardial injury remains prevalent in the increasingly elderly surgical population because tolerance to ischemia is reduced in aged myocardium [5].

Patients who are difficult to wean from cardiopulmonary bypass (CPB) and those who subsequently deteriorate into a low cardiac output state have mortality rates between 50% and 80%

[6]. In established cardiogenic shock, conventional treatment with inotropes, the intra-aortic balloon pump (IABP), or temporary circulatory support devices has not substantially improved survival. In an analysis of risk factors and outcomes for postcardiotomy mechanical support in 19,985 Cleveland Clinic patients, 0.5% received circulatory support with overall survival of 35% [7]. Included were patients who were converted to the HeartMate I implantable system and bridged to transplantation with 72% survival. In the absence of the transplant option, more innovative circulatory support strategies are required to improve survival in the postcardiotomy setting.

Mechanisms of postcardiotomy myocardial dysfunction

Efforts to improve surgical results in patients who have heart failure depend on myocardial protection and preservation of contractile function in the postoperative period. The clinical scenario is well known. The patient who has myocardial ischemia or chronically impaired left ventricular function undergoes combined valve and coronary bypass surgery. The ischemic time exceeds 90 minutes and despite myocardial protection with blood cardioplegia, inotropic support is required to separate from CPB. The vasoconstricted patient returns to the intensive care unit with borderline cardiac index and a blood pressure of 110/70 mm Hg. Over the next 4 hours the blood pressure remains acceptable on inotropic support but the urine output dwindles and the ankles are cold. An IABP is deployed, seems to function well, and optimism returns until the blood gases reveal lactic acidosis and a pH of

* Corresponding author. Oxford Heart Centre, John Radcliffe Hospital, Headley Way, Headington, Oxford OX3 9DU, UK.

E-mail address: swestaby@ahf.org.uk (S. Westaby).

1551-7136/07/$ - see front matter © 2007 Published by Elsevier Inc.
doi:10.1016/j.hfc.2007.05.001

7.28. Despite artificially sustained systemic blood pressure, the patient is in cardiogenic shock. Neither escalating inotropic support nor IABP counter-pulsation can increase systemic blood flow or prevent the downward spiral toward renal shutdown and inexorable deterioration in metabolic status. At this stage, some centers have access to temporary mechanical circulatory support systems and may deploy a left (LVAD) or biventricular (BIVAD) assist device. Survival then ranges from 25% to 50%.

The mechanisms of postischemic dysfunction are well defined [8]. After cardiac surgery myocardial stunning may impair contractile function for several days despite normal or near-normal coronary blood flow and oxygen supply [8,9]. Stunning causes transient systolic and diastolic dysfunction but with potential for full recovery. The underlying pathophysiology is less efficient oxygen use by the contractile apparatus. This inefficiency results from impaired calcium handling by the sarcoplasmic reticulum and reduced calcium sensitivity of the contractile proteins [10]. Myocardial oxygen consumption (MVO_2) for excitation–contraction coupling is inappropriately high in stunned myocardium with a decrease in contractile efficiency (energetically inefficient) [11]. Potential mechanisms of persisting dysfunction include uncoupling between substrate metabolism and energy production, accelerated but useless energy consumption, or impaired energy transfer to the contractile proteins. Alterations in the amount of energy required for calcium handling may increase myocardial oxygen consumption and the calcium transport mechanisms of the sarcoplasmic reticulum are impaired [12]. The calcium sensitivity of the myofilaments is also decreased in stunned compared with normal myocardium together with elevated peak intracellular calcium [13]. This delayed cellular recovery results in mechanoenergetic mismatch and impaired systolic and diastolic relaxation. Conductance catheter studies of pressure–volume loops show an increase in diastolic left ventricular stiffness and decreased contractile efficiency [9].

The β-adrenergic receptor system plays an important role in regulating calcium homeostasis and mediating positive myocardial inotropic effects by way of adenylate cyclase (Fig. 1). Stunned myocardium retains the capacity to respond to inotropic support [14]. Inotropic stimulation by way of β-adrenoreceptors or selective inhibition of phosphodiesterase isoenzymes increases the amount of cellular calcium cycled with each beat. Elevated calcium loading of the cytosol and sarcoplasmic reticulum increases calcium transients, contributing to the disproportionate increase in myocardial oxygen requirement [15]. Possible causes of this problem include free radical damage to cell membranes or enzymes, ischemia-reperfusion injury with activation of protease enzymes, and abnormalities of intracellular calcium cycling.

Although inotropic support improves contractile function in stunned myocardium the effects of prolonged inotropy may be damaging. β-Adrenergic agents improve cardiac output at the expense of increased myocardial oxygen consumption (Table 1) [16]. Although systolic function and blood pressure improve, diastolic dysfunction persists and may deteriorate further. Furthermore, inotropic stimulation does not improve ventricular wall dyssynchrony. At the cellular level decreased myocardial oxidative phosphorylation compounds the increase in MVO_2 [17]. The combination of increased MVO_2 and depleted energy reserves during inotropic drive contributes to myocardial dysfunction and may cause irreversible damage. Pressure–volume loop studies suggest that inotropes increase stroke work independent of MVO_2 causing an energy demand in excess of that required by the contractile apparatus [18]. This oxygen wasting effect, demonstrated in several mechanoenergetic studies, impedes myocardial recovery [19,20].

Increased MVO_2 has been demonstrated during norepinephrine, digitalis, glucagon, and calcium infusions, and confirmed using velocity of contraction and tension-time index models [12,21,22]. The uncoupling of myocardial oxygen consumption and mechanical energy output can be explained by several pathologic processes. These include mitochondrial dysfunction, heterogeneous microcirculation, desynchronized contraction, altered excitation contraction coupling, and an increased energy demand for contractile work [23]. Added to this is an increase in arterial fatty acid levels and a shift toward myocardial use of fatty acids by stunned myocardium [24]. This metabolic shift may have a profound effect on the relationship between MVO_2 and left ventricular mechanical energy.

Continued exposure to high levels of catecholamines during the development of myocardial dysfunction leads to chronic β-adrenergic desensitization [25] (Fig. 2). This desensitization results in decreased effectiveness of the β-adrenergic receptor–stimulating inotropic agents in the failing heart. Patients who have poor left

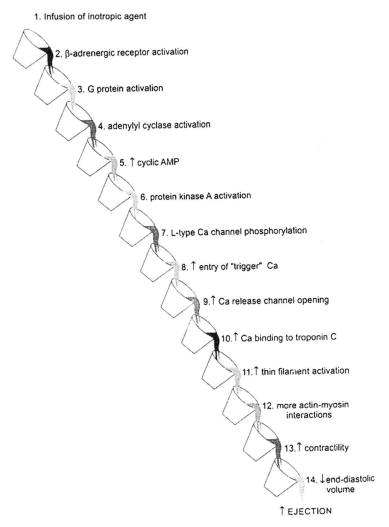

1. Infusion of inotropic agent

2. β-adrenergic receptor activation

3. G protein activation

4. adenylyl cyclase activation

5. ↑ cyclic AMP

6. protein kinase A activation

7. L-type Ca channel phosphorylation

8. ↑ entry of "trigger" Ca

9. ↑ Ca release channel opening

10. ↑ Ca binding to troponin C

11. ↑ thin filament activation

12. more actin-myosin interactions

13. ↑ contractility

14. ↓ end-diastolic volume

↑ EJECTION

Fig. 1. Signal cascade by which adrenergic inotropic agents increase cardiac ejection. At each stop the incoming signal causes the bucket to pour its contents into the next bucket, thereby transmitting the signal down the cascade. In cellular signal transduction different substances pass from one bucket to the next (*From* Katz AM. Physiology of the heart. 3rd edition. Philadelphia: Lippincott/Williams and Wilkins; 2001; with permission.)

ventricular function already have fewer functional β-adrenergic receptors and less responsiveness to inotropic agents. Both α-adrenergic and β-adrenergic receptor numbers and distribution play a role in the outcome of coronary bypass surgery and in the response to revascularization in hibernating myocardium [26]. A decline in β-adrenergic receptor function and receptor density also occurs in patients who have dilated cardiomyopathy [27]. Reversible myocardial β-adrenergic receptor desensitization occurs acutely in the presence of high levels of catecholamines released during

CPB [28]. Myocardial unloading with an LVAD is known to reverse this down-regulation of receptors in failing hearts [29]. This process results in an improved myocardial response to sympathetic stimulation in mechanically unloaded ventricles.

Identification of patients at risk for postoperative low cardiac output syndrome

Coronary and valve patients who have very poor ventricular function often have the most to

Table 1
Pharmacologic properties of frequently used inotropic agents

Pharmacologic properties and therapeutic considerations in using inotropic agents

| Pharmacologic feature | Dobutamine | Milrinone | Dopamine | | Norepinephrine |
			Low dose	High dose	
Receptor agonism					
α	+	0	+	+++	++++
β₁	++++	0	+	++	+
β₂	++	0	0	0	0
Dopaminergic	0	0	+++	++	0
Systemic vascular resistance	↓↓	↓↓↓	↓	↑↑	↑↑↑↑
Stroke volume and cardiac output	↑↑↑↑	↑↑↑↑	↑	↑↑	↑
Ability to increase systemic blood pressure	→ to ↑	→ to ↑	→	↑↑↑	↑↑↑↑
Ventricular filling pressure	↓↓	↓↓↓	↓ to →	→ to ↑↑	→ to ↑↑
Chronotropic	→ to ↑↑	→↓↑	→	→ to ↑↑↑	→ to ↑
Myocardial oxygen demand or supply	→ to ↑	→↓↓	→	→ to ↑↑	→↑↑
Phosphodiesterase inhibitor					

gain from a successful operation. This group is also at greatest risk for postischemic myocardial dysfunction. Because risk-scoring systems provide insufficient weight to very poor ventricular function, some patients may be declined surgery on the grounds of elevated risk [30]. Surgical league tables and report cards inevitably cause surgeons to protect their reputations by avoiding mortality [31]. Paradoxically, refined operative techniques and myocardial protection should widen the availability of surgical repair to high-risk groups. Improved processes are needed to identify very high-risk patients and improve their survival.

The Toronto Hospital Group has defined postoperative low cardiac output syndrome as "the requirement for IABP counter-pulsation or inotropic support for longer than 30 minutes after the patient is returned to the intensive care unit to maintain a systolic blood pressure higher than 90 mm Hg and cardiac index greater than 2.2 L/min/m² " [32]. In a series of several thousand patients the incidence was 9.1% and hospital mortality was 16.9% versus 0.9% ($P < .001$) for those who had an uncomplicated postoperative course. Overall coronary mortality was 2.4%. Analysis of patients in whom low cardiac output syndrome developed showed them to have longer CPB and aortic cross-clamp times, longer postoperative intensive care unit stay, more days of ventilatory support, a longer hospital stay, and a higher

postoperative creatine kinase MB level. They were also more likely to have had a perioperative myocardial infarction (14.3% versus 1.8%, $P < .001$). Patients who had low cardiac output syndrome had a greater mean age (64 versus 61 years, $P < .001$) and had more extensive coronary artery disease ($P < .001$). The operative mortality rate for patients who had complete myocardial revascularization was 2.3% compared with 3.9% in patients in whom revascularization was incomplete ($P = .068$). The prevalence of low cardiac output syndrome was 8.1% after complete revascularization versus 14.6% for others ($P < .001$). Stepwise logistic regression analyses identified nine independent predictors of postoperative low cardiac output syndrome. These were (1) left ventricular ejection fraction less than 20%, (2) repeat operation, (3) emergency operation, (4) female gender, (5) diabetes, (6) age older than 70 years, (7) left main coronary artery disease, (8) recent myocardial infarction, and (9) triple vessel disease. The incidence of postoperative low cardiac output syndrome and the factor-adjusted odds ratio (OR) associated with each predictor were (1) 27%, OR 5.7; (2) 25%, or 4.4; (3) 37%, OR 3.7; (4) 16%, OR 2.5; (5) 13%, OR 1.6; (6) 13%, OR 1.5; (7) 12%, OR 1.4; (8) 16%, OR 1.4; (9) 10%, OR 1.3, respectively.

Poor left ventricular function is the most important index of mortality because these patients have less margin for recovery from post-operative stunning.

Aspects of myocardial protection

Although a detailed review of myocardial protection is beyond the scope of this article, a few important aspects deserve emphasis in the context of the high-risk patient.

There is now compelling evidence that blood cardioplegia decreases myocardial injury during the aortic cross-clamp period and that this conveys significant benefit in high-risk patients. In patients undergoing emergency surgery for unstable angina, Tomasco and colleagues [33] showed that the risk for mortality rose sharply as ejection fraction decreased in patients receiving crystalloid cardioplegia, but that left ventricular function could not be related to mortality when blood cardioplegia was used. Information from a large group of patients in the coronary artery bypass graft (CABG) Patch trial supports these findings [34]. This study was primarily designed to assess the benefits of implanting a cardioverter defibrillator at the time of coronary bypass in patients who had an LVEF less than 36%. Although the patients were not randomized to the type of cardioplegic solution, early outcome could be compared between 190 patients receiving cold crystalloid cardioplegia versus 695 patients who had blood cardioplegia. The crystalloid cardioplegia patients had significantly more operative deaths (2% versus 0.3%, $P = .02$), postoperative Q-wave myocardial infarctions (10% versus 2%, $P < .001$), postcardiotomy low cardiac output syndrome (13% versus 7%, $P = .013$), and postoperative conduction defects (21.6% versus 12.4%, $P = .001$). These results occurred despite blood cardioplegia patients having significantly more risk factors, including diabetes, hypertension, and long cross-clamping time. In patients who had LVEF less than 40%, Ibrahim and colleagues [35] showed blood-based cardioplegic solutions to significantly improve the rate of recovery of myocardial function when compared with crystalloid St Thomas' solution. Consistent with this finding, Kalawski and colleagues [36,37] showed that blood cardioplegia reduced post-reperfusion production of neutrophil-derived superoxide radicals and neutrophil-integrin expression compared with crystalloid cardioplegia.

Although the introduction of warm blood cardioplegia was regarded as a major advance in myocardial protection, numerous experimental and clinical studies to compare cold versus warm blood cardioplegia have failed to establish the superiority of one technique over the other. Inhomogeneous cardioplegia delivery or cold injury may exacerbate perioperative ischemia. Although cold cardioplegia reduces myocardial oxygen consumption and lactate production, it delays the recovery of oxidative metabolism and contractile function [38]. Cold cardioplegia provides better protection in areas that are difficult to perfuse because of coronary obstruction, whereas warm cardioplegia may help to resuscitate the ischemic myocardium [39]. Continuous oxygenated perfusion of the normothermic arrested heart theoretically enables the perfect matching of energy demand and supply so that ischemia is eliminated. The Warm Heart Investigators Trial randomized more than 1700 patients to cold blood or warm blood cardioplegia and showed the latter to result in significantly fewer perioperative myocardial infarctions and cases of low output syndrome [40]. This benefit was evenly distributed across all risk groups. Consistent with these findings an analysis of aggregated data from several clinical trials supports a protective effect of warm-blood cardioplegia given in a continuous fashion [41]. In a large nonrandomized series of 6064 coronary bypass patients, warm blood cardioplegia was associated with better event-free late survival than was cold blood cardioplegia [42]. Prolonged reperfusion with a terminal "hot shot" of cardioplegic solution may help restore function in patients who have poor ventricular function [43].

For patients who have multiple occluded native coronary arteries or extensive disease in previous vein grafts, retrograde delivery of cardioplegia, either alone or in combination with antegrade perfusion, has the capacity to prevent cardioplegia maldistribution and avoid myocardial ischemia [44]. Kaul and colleagues [45] identified the nonuse of coronary sinus cardioplegia as a significant predictor of increased early mortality in patients who had an LVEF less than 20%. This finding was reinforced by the CABG Patch trial data, which showed that the combination of antegrade and retrograde cardioplegia delivery results in less inotrope and IABP use in patients who have LVEF less than 36% than does antegrade cardioplegia alone [34]. Patients in the combined group also show a reduced incidence of postoperative right ventricular dysfunction. In a large series (744 patients) of patients undergoing reoperative coronary bypass, multivariant logistic regression analysis identified failure to use

164   WESTABY et al

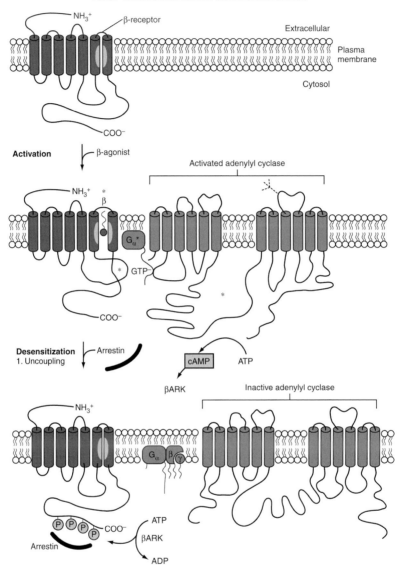

Fig. 2. Mechanisms by which prolonged activation can down-regulate β-adrenergic receptors. Binding of the β agonist to its receptor stimulates adenylyl cyclase to produce cyclic adenosine monophosphate (cAMP). If activation is sustained it causes desensitization by three steps. (*1*) Uncoupling occurs when cAMP stimulates a cAMP-dependent protein kinase called β-adrenergic receptor kinase (bARK), which phosphorylates the β receptor. (*2*) The phosphorylated receptor (*P*) then binds arrestin, an inhibitor protein that prevents further interaction of the receptor with G proteins. Uncoupling is followed by internalization, a reversible process that occurs when the phosphorylated receptor-arrestin complex becomes detached from the plasma membrane and moves to the cytosol. (*3*) The internalized receptors then undergo one of two further reactions. Loss of receptors occurs when β-adrenergic stimulation is continued. This process occurs through irreversible proteolytic digestion of the internalized receptors. Alternatively, inotrope stimulation ends before the internalized receptors are destroyed. The receptors are then dephosphorylated by a phosphoprotein phosphatase, which causes arrestin to dissociate and the receptors to return to the plasma membrane. (*Adapted from* Katz AM. Physiology of the heart. 2nd edition. New York: Raven Press; 1992; with permission.)

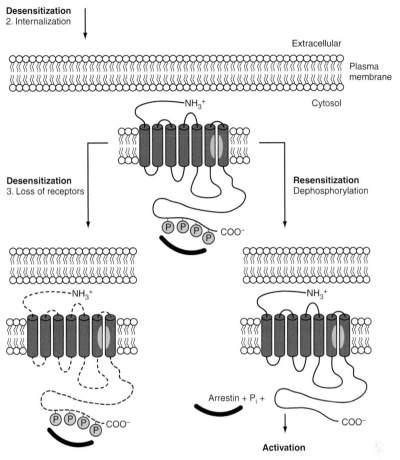

Fig. 2 (*continued*)

retrograde cardioplegic delivery as the strongest independent predictor of in-hospital mortality [46].

Warm cardioplegia may resuscitate ischemic myocardium if it can be delivered uniformly but intermittent discontinuation to permit visualization of distal anastomoses can result in ischemic anaerobic metabolism [47]. The Toronto Group has reported that blood cardioplegia at 29°C (so-called "tepid cardioplegia") can reduce lactate acid production compared with warm (37°C) cardioplegia. This treatment resulted in better contractile function compared with cold (10°C) blood cardioplegia [48]. Others have suggested that patients who have unstable angina or prolonged preoperative ischemia may deplete metabolic reserves and benefit from substrate-enhanced cardioplegia with Krebs Cycle intermediates, such as glutamate, malate, succinate, or fumarate [49]. Patients who have diabetes have diffuse atherosclerotic disease, which may limit cardioplegic distribution and prevent complete revascularization. Some authors therefore recommend both antegrade and retrograde infusions [50]. The rationale is that the different approaches perfuse different myocardial territories and that the combination may provide more homogeneous cardioplegia delivery.

The management of patients at risk for low cardiac output syndrome

Three categories of patients are at substantial risk. First are those who present urgently for surgery, already in cardiogenic shock, often with a complication of myocardial infarction or infective endocarditis. Second is the group submitted for high-risk nontransplant heart failure surgery who have LVEF less than 20% together with renal impairment or aortoiliac disease, which precludes the use of an IABP. The third category includes patients who sustain an unanticipated negative event during surgery, which may prejudice separation from CPB.

Conventional postcardiotomy supportive treatment begins with inotropic drugs, although prolonged use may augment perioperative ischemic injury. Drugs commonly used are dopamine hydrochloride, dobutamine hydrochloride, the inodilator milrinone, and epinephrine. These agents increase stroke work, left ventricular wall tension, and myocardial oxygen consumption, thus depleting energy reserves [51]. High doses may cause endocardial necrosis and impaired diastolic function with an overall negative effect on myocardial recovery. Because of this an IABP or circulatory support system is preferable for patients who have moderate to severe hemodynamic compromise.

Approximately 70,000 IABPs are used annually in the United States with an increasing trend to insert the device preoperatively. The principle effects of the IABP are to reduce left ventricular afterload (and MVO_2), improve diastolic coronary blood flow, and thereby enhance subendocardial perfusion in patients who have elevated left ventricular end diastolic pressure (LVEDP) [52]. The IABP itself does not substantially increase systemic blood flow. Transesophageal echocardiography indicates that peak diastolic coronary flow velocity increases by a mean of 117% with an increase in mean flow velocity integral of 87% [53]. Blood flow velocities of 1.5 to 2.0 times baseline have been measured in the stenosed left anterior descending coronary arteries of patients supported by an IABP [54]. Factors that determine the effectiveness of IABP support include balloon volume, location in the aorta, rate of inflation and deflation, and synchrony relative to the events of the cardiac cycle [55]. The optimal inflation timing has been shown to be slightly preceding the dicrotic notch with deflation bordering on isovolumetric systole. Modern IABP controllers are designed to optimize timing during sinus rhythm and in the presence of cardiac arrhythmias. The IABP also has the capacity to improve right heart function through ventricular interdependence mechanisms and augmentation of right coronary blood flow [56].

Between 10% and 15% of patients undergoing cardiac surgery now receive an IABP either preoperatively to reduce risk or postoperatively after weaning difficulties. Preoperative IABP placement allows stabilization of patients who have acute coronary syndromes before revascularization. In one series of patients who had coronary artery bypass with ejection fraction less than 25%, 30-day mortality with preoperative IABP placement was 2.7% compared with 11.9% for unsupported patients [57]. Baldwin and colleagues [58] developed a model for predicting postcardiotomy IABP survival for patients who required assistance during weaning from CPB. The overall mortality was 48%. If present before or within 10 minutes of the first attempt at weaning from CPB, the following variables were predictors of mortality: (a) complete heart block and the need for pacing, (b) advanced age, (c) elevated preoperative blood urea nitrogen, and (d) female gender. Christenson [59] reported 48% mortality for patients who had IABP who had postcardiotomy heart failure. They identified preoperative myocardial ischemia and combined cardiac surgical procedures as risk factors for mortality.

In a large series of patients who had IABP from the Massachusetts General Hospital, multivariate predictors of death in medical and surgical patients included (a) IABP insertion in the operating room or intensive care unit, (b) transthoracic insertion, (c) advanced age, (d) procedures other than coronary bypass grafting, or (e) percutaneous transluminal coronary angioplasty and insertion for cardiogenic shock [60]. In this series predictors of death were great age, mitral valve replacement, prolonged CPB, urgent or emergency operation, preoperative renal dysfunction, complex ventricular dysrhythmias, right ventricular failure, and emergency resumption of CPB. In the Benchmark Registry and Society of Thoracic Surgeons (USA) National Databases IABP procedures were initiated preoperatively in 52.4% and 63.5%, respectively, of all IABP procedures [61,62]. Preoperative insertion was associated with a mortality of 18.8% to 19.6%, intraoperative insertion 27.6% to 32.3%, and postoperative insertion 39% to 40.5%. There is thus a consensus of opinion that preemptive use of the IABP reduces mortality. The absolute risk reduction is around 7%.

Vascular complications are the most frequent cause of morbidity for patients who have IABP who have rates between 9% and 36% [63]. Femoral cannulation may be complicated by leg ischemia caused by mechanical occlusion, thrombosis, or embolism. Factors predisposing to leg ischemia include female gender, diabetes mellitus, and pre-existing peripheral vascular disease. Possible injuries to the aorta include intramural hematoma, dissection, arterial perforation, and arterial thrombus and embolism. Patients at greatest risk for ischemic complications are those who have a history of peripheral vascular disease, preoperative cardiogenic shock, and a history of smoking. The IABP may also cause mesenteric ischemia or acute pancreatitis, probably as a result of atheroemboli in the celiac axis. Neurologic complications are much less frequent than vascular complications but paraplegia can occur secondary to aortic dissection or adventitial hematoma producing spinal cord infarction. Stroke has occurred after balloon rupture and cerebral helium embolization. Rupture may result in balloon entrapment because blood leaks into the system and forms clots, which block full deflation.

It is important to define which patients will achieve the most benefit from elective IABP use. Reports from the literature indicate that hospital mortality rate for coronary bypass patients who have LVEF less than 25% ranges from 4.8% to 14.3% [64,65]. Wechsler [66] showed that poor LVEF, advanced age, presence of mitral regurgitation, and left main coronary artery disease were risk factors for hospital mortality in patients who had coronary bypass. Dietl [57] showed LVEF less than 25%, repeat CABG, New York Heart Association (NYHA) functional class III or IV, left main coronary disease, urgent or emergency CABG, and LVEDP greater than 20 mm Hg to be indicators of increased hospital mortality. With the growth of percutaneous techniques for less extensive coronary disease, these patient characteristics are becoming more frequent in the surgical setting [67]. As a result the use of the IABP is becoming more frequent. Baskett [68] reported a multicenter comparison of IABP use between 1995 and 2000 that included 29,961 patients. A total of 8.9% received an IABP. Preoperative insertion occurred in 6.3% in contrast to intra- or postoperative insertion in 2.6%. The frequency of IABP use increased from 7% to 10.3% during the 6-year period. Preoperative insertion increased from 5.4% to 7.8%. The rate of IABP use per center varied substantially from 5.9% of patients to 16.4%. A multicenter experience from Alabama reported no survival advantage for prophylactic IABP use in hemodynamically stable high-risk patients, although hospital stay was significantly shorter [69].

Inhaled nitric oxide gas and elevated pulmonary vascular resistance

Pulmonary vascular resistance (PVR) is the primary clinical determinant of right ventricular afterload and an important cause of right ventricular failure and low cardiac output syndrome in high-risk cases. Intravenous drugs, including sodium nitroprusside, nitroglycerine, dobutamine phosphodiesterase inhibitors, and prostaglandin E1, are used clinically as pulmonary vasodilators, but cause vasodilatation and hypotension in the systemic circulation. Hypotension may then impair coronary perfusion pressure and precipitate right ventricular ischemia and failure in the face of elevated PVR. Increased levels of circulating or local vasoconstricting agents released during CPB also contribute to increased pulmonary vascular tone during cardiac surgery. Vascular endothelial cell dysfunction may contribute to pulmonary vasoconstriction following CPB and endothelium-dependent pulmonary vasorelaxation is known to be impaired by CPB [70]. Patients who have elevated pulmonary artery pressure preoperatively are susceptible to acute pulmonary hypertension in the postoperative period.

Inhaled nitric oxide (NO) is a selective pulmonary vasodilator [71]. Once inhaled into the alveolus it diffuses across the alveolar-capillary membrane and into vascular smooth muscle cells. Here NO stimulates guanylate cyclase to generate cyclic guanosine 3, 5-monophosphate (cGMP). In turn cGMP activates protein kinase G, which lowers intracellular calcium causing vascular smooth muscle relaxation. As NO diffuses through the vascular smooth muscle cell and into blood, it is immediately bound to hemoglobin and inactivated. The affinity of hemoglobin for NO is 3000 times greater than for oxygen. By binding to hemoglobin the vasodilating actions of inhaled NO are limited to the pulmonary circulation so that unwanted systemic vasodilation is avoided. In addition the vasodilating action of NO rapidly ceases when the gas is turned off because the half-life of cGMP is less than one minute.

Inhaled NO is clinically administered in concentrations of 1 to 80 ppm. To minimize the potential for toxicity by conversion to NO_2 and nitric acid, it is advisable to monitor the concentrations of inhaled NO and exhaled NO_2 continuously. The lowest possible inhaled oxygen concentration should be used to attenuate the conversion of NO to NO_2. Once bound to hemoglobin NO is converted to methemoglobin, which is unable to bind oxygen. Symptoms of hypoxemia may occur as the concentration of methemoglobin increases beyond 20%. This development is of greater concern during use in infancy than for adult cardiac surgical patients.

In a study of adult patients who had coronary artery bypass inhaled NO produced a consistent reduction in pulmonary arterial pressure and PVR without influencing systemic arterial pressure or systemic vascular resistance [72]. Mean pulmonary arterial pressure was lowered from 29 ± 1 to 21 ± 1 mm Hg. Pulmonary vascular resistance was lowered from 343 ± 30 to 233 ± 25 dyne $\cdot$ s/cm^5 with no change in SVR. Pulmonary vasodilatation with NO 20 ppm produced a significant reduction in transpulmonary gradient and right ventricular stroke work index. Raised PVR is of greater significance in patients who have pulmonary hypertension and valvular heart disease. Patients who have longstanding aortic or mitral valve disease have increased left atrial pressure transmitted retrogradely into the pulmonary arterial circulation. Remodeling of the pulmonary vasculature occurs in response to chronic pulmonary venous obstruction. In addition pulmonary arterial vasoconstriction may occur as a reaction to hypoxia. After left atrial pressure is reduced by valve repair or replacement, increased PVR takes several days or weeks to return to normal levels. For this reason pulmonary vasodilator therapy is useful in patients who have pulmonary hypertension undergoing valve surgery and inhaled NO is the most effective agent.

Clinical experience has been less encouraging than expected. In a small group of patients who had mean preoperative pulmonary arterial pressure of 49 ± 16 mm Hg, Girard reported only a modest reduction to 41 mm Hg after mitral valve replacement and then to 37 mm with inhaled NO at 40 ppm [73]. The modest 9% reduction may reflect irreversible structural changes in response to chronic pulmonary venous outflow obstruction in mitral stenosis. Others have found no response to NO following valve replacement in patients who had valvular heart disease [74,75]. In contrast, patients who had pulmonary hypertension undergoing CABG and serving as controls manifested a 24% decrease in mean pulmonary artery pressure (33 ± 1 to 25 ± 1 mm Hg) together with a 36% fall in PVR (375 ± 30 to 250 ± 30 dyne $\cdot$ s/cm^5) and no change in systemic arterial blood pressure.

Pulmonary vascular tone is believed to be closely related to intracellular levels of vascular smooth muscle cGMP. The net intracellular concentration of cGMP is determined by the balance of its production by guanylate cyclase and degradation by phosphodiesterase (PDE). In cardiac surgical patients whose pulmonary hypertension fails to respond to inhaled NO the effectiveness of inhaled NO can be increased by preventing the breakdown of cGMP by inhibiting PDE with dipyridamole. In a study of 10 cardiac surgical patients who had pulmonary hypertension from aortic and/or mitral valve disease studied in the operating room after valve replacement, neither inhaled NO (40 ppm) alone nor dipyridamole (0.2 mg/kg intravenously) alone lowered PVR or pulmonary artery pressure [76]. The combination of inhaled NO plus dipyridamole effectively produced significant pulmonary vasodilatation, however, thereby converting nonresponding patients into responders. This conversion increased cardiac output by decreasing PVR and mean pulmonary artery pressure without a change in systemic pressure. Combined therapy may benefit patients who have right heart dysfunction by lowering right ventricular afterload.

The function of LVADs depends on transpulmonary blood flow and filling of the prosthetic ventricle. LVAD flow may be compromised if increased PVR limits the ability of the right ventricle to pump blood through the lungs. The pulmonary vasodilating action of inhaled NO has been effectively used in patients who have heart failure to optimize LVAD filling and systemic flow. In patients who had LVAD who were randomly allocated to receive NO (20 ppm) or placebo (nitrogen gas) mean pulmonary artery pressure immediately fell from 35 ± 6 mm Hg to 24 ± 4 mm Hg in patients receiving NO, resulting in an increased LVAD flow from 1.9 ± 0.2 to 2.7 ± 0.3 L/min/m^2 [77]. The placebo had no effect on hemodynamics. When crossed over from nitrogen gas to nitric oxide, control patients responded in a similar way. All patients were weaned from NO within 7 days when LVAD support was sufficient.

Because increased PVR is a risk factor for death following cardiac transplantation, inhaled NO has been used in two important roles. The first is to assess the reactive component of PVR during the pretransplant evaluation. The second is to lower PVR in the early postoperative period following transplantation [78].

Indications and patient selection for circulatory support

A wide variety of temporary and long-term mechanical support devices are now available in affluent health care systems. Blood pumps resuscitate an ever-increasing number of patients who have heart failure by LVAD or BIVAD support with or without cardiac transplantation. The goal of postcardiotomy circulatory support is to restore normal hemodynamics and oxygen delivery in patients in whom the native heart is temporarily unable to sustain this function despite IABP and inotropic support. Accepted criteria for circulatory support in cardiogenic shock include a cardiac index less than 2.0 L/min/m^2, systolic blood pressure less than 90 mm Hg, and pulmonary capillary wedge pressure greater than 20 mm Hg with biochemical evidence of poor tissue perfusion (reflected by increasing serum creatinine and liver transaminases) [79]. The patient is usually oliguric and acidotic with cool extremities and obtunded mental state. In the face of maximum supportive treatment these are indices of impending death. Only one third of patients recover irrespective of mechanical circulatory support. This finding indicates that the traditional guidelines for LVAD or BIVAD deployment should be revised to promote earlier intervention now that safer, more user-friendly devices are emerging.

Patient selection is crucial in determining a successful outcome. The presence of irreversible renal, hepatic, or respiratory failure remains an absolute contraindication to initiating support. Established stroke and sepsis are relative contraindications. Data from the American International Society of Heart and Lung Transplantation Registry indicate that patients older than 70 years of age have decreased survival after circulatory support, although weaning is not affected by age [80]. Risk stratification models show the need for mechanical ventilation, urine output less than 30 mL/h, preoperative central venous pressure greater than 16 mm Hg, hepatic dysfunction (prothrombin time >16 seconds), and increasing serum creatinine and bilirubin levels to be adverse prognostic risk factors [81].

There are currently two groups of patients in whom temporary support is beneficial and for whom Food and Drug Administration (FDA)–approved devices exist. The first includes those patients who sustain reversible myocardial injury with a reasonable expectation of myocardial recovery and device removal in less than 2 weeks. Along with postcardiotomy failure, this group includes patients who have acute myocardial infarction and viral myocarditis. Extracorporeal pulsatile and nonpulsatile ventricular assist devices (VADs) and extracorporeal membrane oxygenation are used in these patients. The second group includes those in whom recovery is unlikely and who require bridge to cardiac transplantation. Limited-duration extracorporeal systems and implantable LVADs are used in the bridge to transplant setting. In addition to these conventional approaches, long-term bridge to myocardial recovery (by ventricular remodeling) in chronic heart failure and short-term bridge to a long-term implantable LVAD are emerging indications for circulatory support [82].

The time of initiation of postcardiotomy support has a profound effect on outcome. Early deployment based on predictive models (derived from hemodynamic parameters and level of intraoperative inotropic support) provide improved rates of weaning and survival to hospital discharge [83]. Delay increases the need for biventricular support, which is associated with decreased survival. As the severity of cardiogenic shock and organ dysfunction increase so does the need for biventricular support. An episode of cardiac arrest before support decreases survival from around 47% to 7% [84]. Data from the Abiomed BV 5000 Registry show that delay in initiating support for more than 6 hours after weaning from CPB is associated with decreased survival (44% versus 14%) [85]. If a patient is weaned from CPB on two high-dose inotropes, the hospital mortality is around 42%. This rate increases to 80% if three high-dose inotropes are required to separate from CPB. If VAD insertion occurs within 3 hours of the first attempt to wean from CPB, then 60% can be separated from VAD support with 43% hospital discharge rate. This finding contrasts with only 27% VAD separation and 7% hospital discharge when VAD insertion is delayed for more than 3 hours after weaning from CPB [86].

Pulsatile extracorporeal circulatory support systems

In the 1980s arterial pulse pressure was believed to be an important component of human circulation. Strenuous efforts were made to develop pulsatile blood pumps for CBP. Introduced clinically in 1982, the Thoratec VAD (Thoratec Corporation, Berkley CA, USA) is an external pulsatile pneumatic system that offers left, right, or biventricular support [87]. The pump's polycarbonate housing contains a flexible, seamless, segmented polyurethane sac. Mechanical tilting disc valve prosthesis in the inlet and outlet cannulas provides one-way flow (Fig. 3). For left ventricular support the inflow cannula is placed in the left atrium or left ventricular apex and the outflow cannula is inserted into the ascending aorta by way of a Dacron graft. For right ventricular support the inflow and outflow cannulas are placed in the right atrium and pulmonary artery, respectively. The tubing exits from the skin subcostally and the cannulas enter the blood pump, which rests against the abdomen (see Fig. 3). In a newer version, the pumps can be implanted under the abdominal subcutaneous tissue for longer-term support. The external console provides alternating positive and negative pressure to the pump by way of a pneumatic driveline. To maintain physiologic blood flow the volume (fill-to-empty) mode of operation allows the pump to change speed as needed. Three pumping modes are available: (a) fixed-rate mode depends on a preset pattern independent of the patient's natural heart rate, (b) synchronous mode is attuned to the patient's ECG so that the flow ejection is triggered by the R wave, (c) a synchronous fill-to-empty mode provides continuous maximal flow regulated by the pump's filling rate. For patients who need biventricular support, excessive pulmonary congestion is prevented by adjusting right-sided flow so that it is slightly less than left-sided flow.

Because of the long-established safety record and versatility, the Thoratec system is used widely for support in critically ill patients as a bridge to either transplantation or cardiac recovery. Drawbacks include limited patient mobility and the need for external cannulas. To prevent thrombus formation within the pump sac, patients must undergo continuous anticoagulation. Although the device can be used for adult patients who have a wide range of body size (body surface area 0.73–2.5 m^2) it is too large for pediatric support. Similar extracorporeal pneumatic devices, such as the Berlin Excor (Fig. 4) and Medos systems, have been scaled down for use in infants and children [88,89].

In one large multicenter study, 74% of Thoratec LVAD patients and 58% of BIVAD patients survived to transplantation with a hospital discharge rate of 89% and 81%, respectively [90].

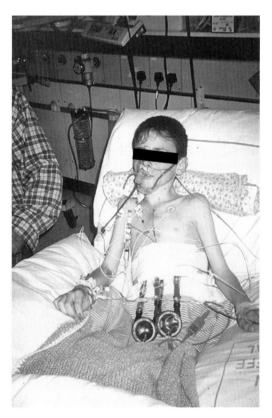

Fig. 4. The Berlin Excor system supporting a child who has end-stage idiopathic dilated cardiomyopathy, pending cardiac transplantation.

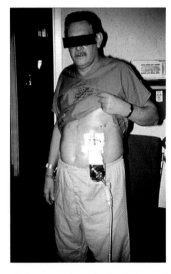

Fig. 3. Ambulatory patient who has left ventricular support with the Thoratec VAD.

The most common complications were bleeding (42%), infection (36%), renal failure (35%), hepatic failure (24%), hemolysis (19%), respiratory failure (17%), multiorgan failure (16%), and neurologic events (22%). It may be difficult to predict which patients will need biventricular support. Those who have clinically severe right heart failure, elevated pulmonary vascular resistance, and intractable ventricular dysrhythmias are most likely to require a right ventricular assist device because systemic venous return increases further during LVAD support. The Berlin Heart and Medos systems use similar cannula connections and have also been used for prolonged (weeks or months) bridge to transplantation or recovery.

The Abiomed BVS 5000 was the first cardiac assist device approved by the FDA (1992) for postcardiotomy patients [91]. After the IABP it has been the second most popular system used in more than 4000 patients. The BVS 5000 (Fig. 5) is an external pulsatile assist device that is capable of providing short-term left, right, or biventricular support. Although designed for a maximum use of 2 weeks, it has been successfully used in transplant candidates for much longer periods. The system components include transthoracic cannulas, disposable external pumps, and a microprocessor-controlled pneumatic drive console. Each pump has an upper chamber (atrium) that collects blood by means of gravity and a lower chamber (ventricle) that propels blood out of the pump. Two trileaflet valves, one located between the two chambers and the other located in the outflow portion of the lower chamber, produce one-way flow. Blood drains from the collecting chamber into the blood pump by gravity. This passive filling avoids native atrial collapse, inflow cannula suction of air, and hemolysis. Each chamber contains a smooth-surfaced 100 mL polyurethane bladder. Compressed air enters the blood pump's ventricular chamber during pump systole, causing bladder collapse and thus returning the blood to the patient. During diastole air is vented through the console through the atmosphere allowing ventricular bladder filling. A single system supports one side of the heart. The collecting bladders operate in a fill-to-empty mode. Adequate intravascular volume is mandatory for optimal device flow. Inadequate filling occurs if the external blood pump position is too high, whereas prolonged filling may occur if the blood pump position is too low or if the patient is volume overloaded.

Depending on the type of support required, the inflow cannulas are placed in the right and/or left atrium. The outflow cannulas are anastomosed to the pulmonary artery or the aorta by way of a Dacron graft. The cannulas exit from the patient

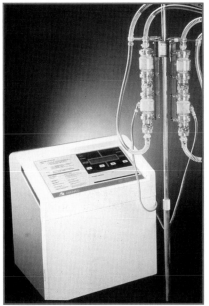
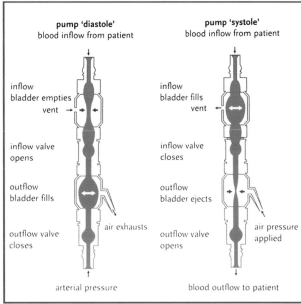

Fig. 5. The ABIOMED BVS 5000 pumping system.

subcostally and are covered with Dacron velour at
the exit sites, which permits sternal closure. Power
is supplied by way of the pneumatic drive console,
which is connected to the lower chamber by
means of a driveline. The console automatically
maintains the stroke volume at 82 mL and
monitors passing filling, thereby adjusting the
pump rate as needed to provide flows of up to
4 L/min. Pumping is not synchronized with the
patient's own heart. The automated control system automatically adjusts for changes in the
patient's preload and afterload and requires
minimal operator intervention. This simplicity
renders the device easier for nurses to manage
than an IABP.

The two-valve design mimics a natural heart
and fully decompresses the ventricle while providing pulsatile flow at physiologic levels to the
major organs, which allows withdrawal of inotropes to reduce myocardial oxygen demand. The
mechanism is afterload sensitive so that the outflow graft must not be kinked or impaired.
Implantation is usually performed with the patient still on CPB. The outflow cannulas are
anastomosed first to the main pulmonary artery
and inferolateral aspect of the aorta. Once the
outflow cannulas are inserted the inflow cannulas
are placed in the mid right atrial wall and either
the left atrium or left ventricular apex. The choice
depends on ease of insertion and the presence of
a mitral prosthesis. Left ventricular cannulation is
used if the left atrium is not accessible because of
small size or scarring from previous surgery. If
there is a mechanical mitral prosthesis, left ventricular cannulation is preferred to maintain flow
across the prosthesis and reduce the risk for
thromboembolism.

Once the patient is weaned from CPB and BVS
5000 support has been initiated, the heparin is
reversed to achieve a normal activated clotting
time. All cannulation sites are inspected for
bleeding and then the chest is closed if possible
to maintain body temperature and prevent infection. After bleeding has stopped the pump
requires full anticoagulation as thrombi may
form in the sinuses of the valves. The patient
can then be extubated during support. This device
can be used for all forms of recoverable heart
failure, including acute myocardial infarction,
myocarditis, thoracic trauma, and right ventricular support, when an implantable LVAD is
deployed. If recovery does not occur the pumps
can be used as a bridge to transplantation or an
implantable LVAD for long-term support.

From Abiomed's Worldwide Registry, 63% of
cases have been postcardiotomy patients who had
an average age of 56 years and a mean duration of
5 days' support [91]. A total of 15% had dilated
cardiomyopathy, 7% had acute myocardial infarction, 9% had a failed cardiac transplant, and
6% had myocarditis or other indications. A total
of 52% of patients have biventricular assist, 34%
have left ventricular assist, and 14% have isolated
right ventricular assist. Postcardiotomy support
resulted in 30% survival, whereas the acute myocardial infarction hospital discharge rate was only
33%. When the pumps were inserted within 3
hours of the decision to implant survival was
60% versus 20% when insertion was delayed. Success with left ventricular assist alone was better
with earlier implantation. The longest duration
of support was 90 days.

Extracorporeal centrifugal blood pumps

Centrifugal pumps impart momentum to fluid
by fast-moving blades, impellers, or concentric
cones [92]. Fluid enters the pump axially from an
inlet pipe or tubing and is caught up between veins
or stages and whirled outward (Fig. 6). Rotation
of the impeller causes the velocity of blood to
change while it moves toward the periphery of
the pump. As blood exits through the outlet
port, pressure is increased. Centrifugal pumps
can provide high flow rates with low pressure increases but are particularly sensitive to afterload.
Flow is continuous without pulse pressure. The
major indication for centrifugal mechanical assistance is failure to wean from CPB secondary to
left, right, or biventricular failure. After the first
unsuccessful attempt the heart is allowed more reperfusion time on CPB while it is determined
whether the surgical repair can be improved.
IABP support is instituted. If subsequent weaning
events with high-dose multiple inotropes prove
unsuccessful (and death is imminent), the centrifugal pump is applied for salvage.

Cannulation sites are the same as for pulsatile
blood pumps. The preferred right atrial site is the
junction of the inferior vena cava and right atrium
orientating the tip of a 36F cannula superiorly.
This placement allows the cannula direct exit from
the mediastinum inferiorly through the abdominal
wall without kinking. Flow at any given centrifugal pump speed is preload and afterload dependent. In the absence of adequate preload the
atrium collapses around the inlet cannula and
causes cessation of pump flow. The atrium then

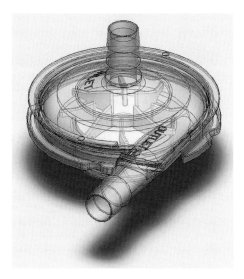
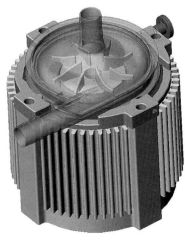

Fig. 6. Centrifugal pump mechanism providing continuous (nonpulsatile) blood flow.

fills but with inadequate volume the process repeats itself rapidly and must be managed by decreasing the RMP or administering fluid to the patient. A sudden decrease in flow may also suggest an abrupt increase in afterload (if the patient wakes up) or a kinked outflow tube. Afterload reduction or correction of the technical problem restores pump flow. In the event of right-sided bypass with pulmonary hypertension, nitric oxide is used to reduce pulmonary vascular resistance.

Incorporation of a hemofiltration system in the tubing circuit is an expedient technique for removal of excess intravascular volume. The ultrafiltration rate is controlled by passing the effluent through an infusion pump that controls the egress and avoids large intravascular volume shifts. Left heart bypass is always started slowly while right heart function is assessed. Increased delivery of blood to the right heart may precipitate right ventricular distension and failure. The centrifugal pump speed is set at the lowest RMP that accomplishes the prescribed flow (3–6 L/min). Central venous pressure is maintained in the physiologic range by addition of blood or fluids.

In the postcardiotomy situation, coagulopathy is common and bleeding can be troublesome. The preferred anticoagulation strategy is to completely reverse heparin with protamine in the operating room and then begin a heparin infusion postoperatively when the partial thromboplastin time (PTT) decreases to less than 60 seconds. This decrease rarely occurs during the first 24 hours. The PTT is then maintained in the range between 40 and 60 seconds. Although it is preferable to close the sternum this must be left open in many cases to avoid cardiac compression and tamponade. If sternal closure is impractical, skin closure is undertaken either by direct apposition or with a transparent silicone sheet sutured to the edges and covered with an adhesive drape to produce an airtight seal. In the event of late tamponade mediastinal exploration is easily performed in the intensive care unit, thereby avoiding a return trip to the operating room. Renal failure or pulmonary edema is managed with the hemofilter.

Because of durability problems the first-generation centrifugal pumps, such as Medtronic Biomedicus, Sarms 3M and St Jude models, are not used for more than 5 days. The system must be supervised by trained personnel and the pump components should be replaced every 48 to 96 hours. In addition the external cannulas pose an infection risk. Despite the risk for heparin-bonded circuits and connectors, the pump's electromagnetic elements are potential sites for thrombus and fibrin formation. To minimize embolic risk and troublesome bleeding through heparinization, the goal is to remove the device as soon as hemodynamic competence and stability return. Weaning from centrifugal mechanical support is straightforward. As left ventricular function recovers, pulse pressure is observed during full flow and amplified as pump speed is decreased. Thermodilution cardiac output measurements allow right ventricular output to be measured. By subtracting pump flow the proportion of cardiac output contributed by the recovering left ventricle can be determined. When a right ventricular index of 2.0 to 2.2 L/m² is obtained with minimal inotropic support and the pump at low flow, on and off trials are performed and repeated every 8 hours until recovery is confirmed. Timing of weaning from biventricular support is more difficult and requires echocardiographic assessment of ventricular function. Pulmonary arterial mixed venous oxygen saturation less than 50% reflects inadequate tissue perfusion. If perfusion is adequate, both devices are temporarily decreased to the lowest RPM that prevents flow reversal, after which on and off trials are observed. In practice there is a finite window of opportunity for device removal between myocardial recovery and device-related complications. Around 50% of patients recover sufficient myocardial function to be weaned, half of whom survive to leave the hospital.

Outcome after circulatory support for postcardiotomy cardiogenic shock

Pae and colleagues [93] from the Pennsylvania State University reviewed combined registry data on the use of first-generation temporary LVADs between 1985 and 1990. A total of 965 patients were treated for postcardiogenic shock, of whom 45% were weaned from the system and 25% were discharged from the hospital. Notably 90% of patients who survived to leave the hospital were weaned from the pump within 1 week. Those requiring univentricular support alone faired better irrespective of whether pulsatile pneumatic or nonpulsatile centrifugal pumps were used. Patient age greater than 70 years was the principle determinant of mortality. Irrespective of multiple complications, including bleeding, stroke, and renal failure, patients who left the hospital had 2-year actuarial survival of 82%, and 86% were in NYHA functional class I or II. In rare instances of device dependency (4.5%) those patients who did not have contraindications to transplantation were sustained until a donor organ became available. Of the transplanted patients, 62% were discharged from the hospital.

Golding and colleagues [94] from the Cleveland Clinic reported a 12-year experience of 91 patients supported with a centrifugal blood pump after failure to wean from CPB. Mean age of postcardiotomy patients was 54.8 years and mean duration of support was 3.56 days (range 1 hour to 19 days). A total of 62% of the patients were successfully weaned but only 25% survived to leave the hospital. Bleeding occurred in 87% with an astonishing mean transfusion requirement of 53 units. Renal failure occurred in 47%, cerebral vascular accident in 13%, thromboembolism in 13%, and hepatic insufficiency in 13%. In the follow-up period one third of patients died but most of the remainder were in NYHA class I or II. Patients who had biventricular failure and renal failure had worse late outcomes.

Lee and colleagues [95] from the Johns Hopkins Hospital performed a retrospective review of 7385 adult patients undergoing cardiac surgery in a 6-year period. Of these 1% developed postcardiotomy cardiogenic shock, around one third of whom met the institutional criteria for circulatory support with a centrifugal blood pump. Mean age of the patients was 50.8 ± 12.9 years (range 22 to 72 years) and mean duration of ventricular assistance was 2.8 ± 2.5 days (range 4 hours to 10 days, median 2 days). Complications included serious bleeding in half of the patients, cardiac tamponade, systemic embolism, seizures, and sepsis. More than half of the patients required re-exploration for bleeding or cardiac tamponade. Some 32% of the patients were discharged from the hospital and were alive and well (NYHA class I or II) 2 years later. In this series older age was a relative contraindication to mechanical support.

Imasaka and colleagues [96] from Kyushu University, Japan, reviewed their experience in 22 mechanically supported patients who had postcardiotomy cardiogenic shock. A total of 41% were successfully weaned and 27% survived to hospital discharge. The duration of circulatory assist ranged from 21 to 211 hours (median 66 hours). In those who could be weaned duration of support was less than 3 days. Major complications were re-exploration for bleeding in 18%, renal dysfunction in 77%, liver dysfunction in 59%, infection in 32%, pulmonary dysfunction in 36%, and cerebral injury in 41%. Oliguria and progressive acidosis were indices of insufficient hemodynamic recovery and predictors for early death. The authors suggested early conversion from temporary support to a long-term implantable LVAD when risk factors suggested poor outcome.

DeRose and colleagues [97] from the Columbia Presbyterian Medical Center, New York, adopted a policy of early implantation of the ThermoCardioSystems HeartMate LVAD (Fig. 7) for patients who developed circulatory failure after high-risk cardiac surgery. In a 4-year period 12 patients received this LVAD for postcardiotomy cardiogenic shock following CABG. The median

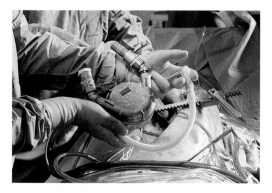

Fig. 7. The TermoCardioSystems HeartMate I LVAD.

time to device insertion was 3.5 days, over which time patients had been managed with inotropic support or an IABP. The mean duration of LVAD support was 103 ± 19 days (range 2–225 days). Of the 12 patients included in the report, 1 recovered sufficiently for device explantation and 9 of the remaining 11 patients (82%) survived to undergo transplantation with successful hospital discharge in each case. The major complication was device-related infection in half of the patients. The authors concluded that long-term outcome after postcardiotomy cardiogenic shock could be markedly improved with the use of an implantable LVAD early in the postoperative course. After this, survival depended on cardiac transplantation before a critical device-related adverse event.

From these and other reports, it is clear that less than one third of patients who suffer postcardiotomy heart failure refractory to the use of the IABP can be salvaged after the onset of cardiogenic shock. Device-related adverse events, particularly bleeding and infection, have so far precluded widespread prophylactic deployment of temporary LVADs for high-risk patients to prevent cardiogenic shock.

Elective transfer from cardiopulmonary bypass to centrifugal blood pump support in very high-risk cardiac surgery

The decision to preemptively deploy an LVAD must balance safety with efficacy. To improve outcome in borderline survival situations following high-risk cardiac surgery the Oxford Group decided to wean directly from CPB to a new temporary centrifugal blood pump designed to reduce bleeding and thromboembolic complications [98]. The rationale for elective LVAD

deployment is straightforward. The failing heart beats more than 120,000 times per day pumping in excess of 7000 L of blood against an increased afterload. A dilated heart has greater wall tension and increased myocardial energy demand but suffers reduced subendocardial blood flow. After surgery ischemia-reperfusion injury may trigger the downward spiral into cardiogenic shock and multiorgan failure. Inotropic agents temporarily elevate systemic blood pressure but they exert deleterious effects by increasing heart rate, afterload, and subendocardial ischemia. In contrast an LVAD unloads the ventricle, boosts coronary and systemic blood flows, and promotes myocardial recovery. Some inotropic support may be required to sustain right ventricular contractility in the face of increased venous return.

The Levitronix Centrimag short-term VAD is an extracorporeal system composed of a single-use centrifugal blood pump, a motor, a console, a flow probe, and a tubing circuit (Fig. 8). The device is composed of a bearingless motor that combines the drive, the magnetic bearing, and the rotor function in a single unit. The motor generates the magnetic bearing force that levitates the rotor into the pump housing while also generating the torque necessary to produce the unidirectional flow. The importance of magnetic levitation is the absence of bearings and seals resulting in minimal friction or heat generation in the blood path. The rotor surface is uniformly washed which minimizes the areas of blood stagnation and turbulence in the pump. To reduce hemolysis the mechanical gaps in the pump are greater than 0.6 mm to allow sheer forces to be low. This device can produce flows up to 10 L/min under normal physiologic conditions with a priming volume of 31 mL. The device is CE mark approved for short-term circulatory support and is commercially available through Europe. Initial European clinical trials in postcardiotomy cardiogenic shock have been encouraging over mean support periods of 2 weeks and the longest support period of 64 days. Overall 30-day mortality was 50%, which compares favorably with that reported for other devices. The system is reliable and versatile so that it can be quickly implemented in situations of rapid deterioration. Device mechanical reliability and relatively low complication rates make the Levitronix pump safe to use for patients who need time for evaluation for cardiac transplantation or a longer-term device.

For elective transfer from CPB to centrifugal blood pump support the patients at highest risk for postcardiotomy cardiogenic shock are

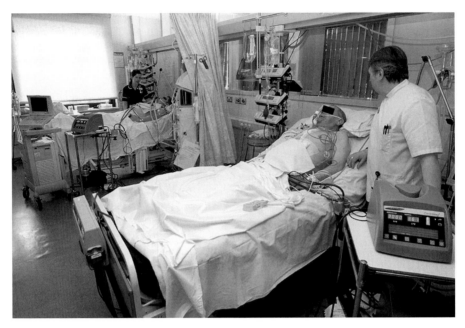

Fig. 8. The Levitronix system supporting two patients in the cardiac intensive care unit.

selected before surgery. Candidates may have chronic left ventricular dysfunction with LVEF less than 20%, recent acute myocardial infarction, impaired renal function, or aortoiliac disease precluding IABP use. LVAD implantation is undertaking during 30 minutes of reperfusion time before discontinuation of CPB. Conduits for the inflow and outflow cannulas

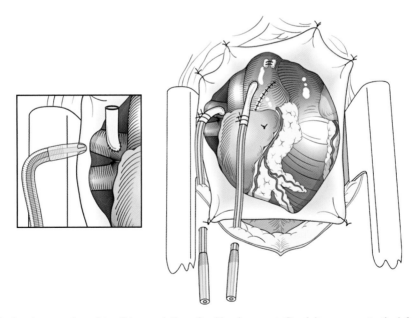

Fig. 9. Method to improve the safety of decannulation after blood support. Conduits are sewn to the left superior pulmonary vein and ascending aorta through which the inflow and outflow cannulas are attached to the heart. (*Adapted from* Westaby S, Balacumaraswami L, Evans BJ, et al. Elective transfer from cardiopulmonary by pass to centrifugal blood pump support in very high-risk cardiac surgery. J Thorac Cardiovasc Surg 2007;133(2):577; with permission. Copyright © 2007, The American Association for Thoracic Surgery.)

are used to improve the safety of decannulation (Fig. 9). A tube of descending aortic homograft (8 cm × 10 mm diameter) is sewn to an incision at the junction of the superior pulmonary vein with the left atrium. Through this conduit is introduced the 32F right-angled wire-reinforced venous cannula into the center of the left atrium. Ligatures are placed around the homograft tube to retain the inflow cannula in position. The distal end of the venous cannula is brought through the skin below the sternotomy wound and then filled by raising left atrial pressure. A Dacron polyester fabric graft (8 mm) is then sewn to the ascending aorta with a side clamp. The straight 22F arterial inflow cannula is inserted through this graft, secured into place by ligatures, and brought out through the skin adjacent to the venous cannula. The system is filled during reperfusion and de-airing of the native heart. The patient is then weaned directly from CPB onto LVAD flow to provide between 3 and 4 L/min. Antegrade cardiac ejection continues to provide systemic pulsatility. Combined output from the device and the native left ventricle is around 3.0 L/min/m^2. Transesophageal echocardiography is used to confirm the position of the inflow cannula and the efficacy of de-airing.

After protamine administration the sternotomy wound is closed to allow extubation during support. To minimize bleeding no anticoagulation is given for 12 hours. Once the chest tube drainage is less than 50 mL/h heparin infusion is given to provide an activated partial thromboplastin time ratio of 1.5 to 2.5. For recovery after ischemic arrest the support duration is usually less than 7 days. In this time frame the Levitronix pump is reliable, safe, and effective. It is readily managed by nursing staff and easily portable. Reoperation for bleeding and decannulation problems are avoided by the use of the conduits.

With a view to explant, myocardial function is assessed daily with the pump flow turned down to 2.0 L/min/m^2. After sustainable improvement in myocardial function has been achieved, the patient is returned to the operating room, the pump is switched off, and the cannulas are withdrawn. The grafts are ligated close to their insertion to prevent thrombus formation. As part of the step-down process an IABP is used for a further 24 to 48 hours.

The elective circulatory support strategy has been used successfully in a small series of patients who had coronary and aortic valve disease, all with LVEF less than 15% [98]. All patients who

had chronic heart failure survived. The only mortality occurred in relation to extensive recent myocardial infarction with ventricular septal defect in which a salvage procedure proved unsuccessful and support was withdrawn because of advanced hepatorenal failure.

To date the Levitronix Centrimag pump has been used in more than 300 patients, of whom 45% of cases have been salvage postcardiotomy support with a mean of 9 days and 53% survival. It is likely that the 47% mortality could have been reduced substantially by anticipating postoperative deterioration and using the blood pump electively to prevent cardiogenic shock during the duration of reversible postischemic stunning.

References

[1] O'Connor GT, Birkmeyer JD, Dacey LJ, et al. Results of a regional study of modes of death associated with coronary artery bypass grafting. Ann Thorac Surg 1998;66:1323–8.

[2] Marso SP, Bhatt DL, Roe MT, et al. Enhanced efficacy of eptifibatide administration in patients with acute coronary syndrome requiring in-hospital coronary artery bypass grafting. Circulation 2000;102:2952–8.

[3] Liu JY, Birkmeyer NJO, Sanders JH. Risks of morbidity and mortality in dialysis patients undergoing coronary artery bypass surgery. Circulation 2000;102:2973–7.

[4] Connolly HM, Oh JK, Schaff HV, et al. Severe aortic stenosis with low transvalvular gradient and severe left ventricular dysfunction: result of aortic valve replacement in 52 patients. Circulation 2000;102:2952–8.

[5] Mariani J, Ou R, Bailey M, et al. Tolerance to ischemia and hypoxia is reduced in aged human myocardium. J Thorac Cardiovasc Surg 2000;120:660–7.

[6] Goldstein DJ, Oz MC. Mechanical support for postcardiotomy cardiogenic shock. Semin Thorac Cardiovasc Surg 2000;12(3):220–8.

[7] Smedira NG, Blackstone EH. Postcardiotomy mechanical support: risk factors and outcomes. Ann Thorac Surg 2001;71(3 Suppl):S60–6.

[8] Bolli R, Marban E. Molecular and cellular mechanisms of myocardial stunning. Physiol Rev 1999;79:609–34.

[9] Bavaria JE, Furukawa S, Kreiner G, et al. Myocardial oxygen utilization after reversible global ischemia. J Thorac Cardiovasc Surg 1990;100:210–20.

[10] Krause SM, Jacobus WE, Becker LC. Alterations in cardiac sarcoplasmic reticulum calcium transport in the postischaemic "stunned" myocardium. Circ Res 1989;65:526–30.

[11] Furukawa S, Bavaria JE, Kreiner G, et al. Relationship between total mechanical energy and oxygen

consumption in the stunned myocardium. Ann Thorac Surg 1990;49:543–8.

[12] Kusuoka H, Koretsune Y, Chacko VP, et al. Excitation-contraction coupling in postischemic myocardium. Does failure of activator Ca^{2+} transients underlie stunning? Circ Res 1990;66:1268–76.

[13] Korvald C, Elvenes OP, Ytrebo LM, et al. Oxygen-wasting effect of inotropy in the "virtual work model". Am J Physiol 1999;276:H1339–45.

[14] Bavaria JE, Furukawa S, Kreiner G, et al. Effect of circulatory assist devices on stunned myocardium. Ann Thorac Surg 1990;49(1):123–8.

[15] Sunderdiek U, Korbmacher B, Gams E, et al. Myocardial efficiency in stunned myocardium. Comparison of Ca^{2+} sensitisation and PDE III—inhibition as energy consumption. Eur J Cardiothorac Surg 2000; 18:83–9.

[16] Ellis SG, Wynne J, Braunwald E, et al. Response of reperfusion-salvaged, stunned myocardium to inotropic stimulation. Am Heart J 1984;107:13–9.

[17] Laxter SB, Becker LC, Ambrosio G, et al. Reduced aerobic metabolic efficiency in globally stunned myocardium. J Mol Cell Cardiol 1989;21:419–26.

[18] Suga H, Hisano R, Goto Y, et al. Effects of positive inotropic agents on the relation between oxygen consumption and systolic pressure volume area in canine left ventricle. Circ Res 1983;53:306–18.

[19] Braunwald E, Kloner RA. The stunned myocardium: prolonged, post-ischemic ventricular dysfunction. Circulation 1992;66:1146–9.

[20] Bolli R. Mechanism of myocardial stunning. Circulation 1990;82:723–38.

[21] Ito BR, Tate H, Kobayashi M, et al. Reversibly injured, postischemic canine myocardium retains normal contractile reserve. Circ Res 1987;61: 834–46.

[22] Myens B, Sergeant P, Wouters P, et al. Mechanical support with microaxial blood pumps for postcardiotomy left ventricular failure: can outcome be predicted? J Thorac Cardiovasc Surg 2000;120: 393–400.

[23] Burkhoff D. Myocardial energetics and the postischemic heart. Ann Thorac Surg 1990;49:525–7.

[24] Liedtke AJ, De Maison L, Eggleston AM, et al. Changes in substrate metabolism and effects of excess fatty acid in reperfused myocardium. Circ Res 1988;62:535–42.

[25] Fowler MB, Laser JA, Hopkins GL, et al. Assessment of the beta-adrenergic receptor pathway in the intact failing human heart: progressive receptor down-regulation and subsensitivity to agonist response. Circulation 1986;74(6):1290–302.

[26] Shan K, Bick RJ, Poindexter BJ, et al. Altered adrenergic receptor density in myocardial hibernation in humans. Circulation 2000;102:2599–606.

[27] Lohse MJ, Engelhardt S, Danner S, et al. Mechanisms of beta-adrenergic receptor desensitisation: from molecular biology to heart failure. Basic Res Cardiol 1996;91(Suppl 2):29–34.

[28] Gerhardt MA, Booth JV, Chesnut LC, et al. Acute desensitisation of myocardial β adrenergic receptors during cardiopulmonary bypass. Circulation 1991; 84:2559–67.

[29] Ogletree-Hughes ML, Stull LB, Sweet WE, et al. Mechanical unloading restores β adrenergic responsiveness and reverses receptor downregulation in the failing human heart. Circulation 2001;104:881–6.

[30] Westaby S. League tables, risk assessment and an opportunity to improve standards. Br J Cardiol (Acute Interv Cardiol) 2002;9:5–10.

[31] Shahian DM, Normand SL, Torchiana DF, et al. Cardiac surgery report cards, comprehensive review and statistical critique. Ann Thorac Surg 1999;68: 1195–202.

[32] Rao V, Ivanov J, Weisel RD, et al. Predictors of low cardiac output syndrome after coronary artery bypass. J Thorac Cardiovasc Surg 1996;112(1):38–51.

[33] Tomasco B, Cappiello A, Fiorilli R, et al. Surgical revascularisation for acute coronary insufficiency: analysis of risk factors for hospital mortality. Ann Thorac Surg 1997;64:678–83.

[34] Flack JE, Cook JR, May SJ, et al. Does cardioplegia type affect outcome and survival in patients with advanced left ventricular dysfunction? Results from the CABG Patch trial. Circulation 2000; 102(19 Suppl 3) 11184–89.

[35] Ibrahim MF, Venn GE, Young CP, et al. A clinical comparative study between crystalloid and blood-based St Thomas' hospital cardioplegic solution. Eur J Cardiothorac Surg 1999;15(1):75–83.

[36] Kalawski R, Balinski M, Bugajski P, et al. Stimulation of neutrophil activation during coronary artery bypass grafting: comparison of crystalloid and blood cardioplegia. Ann Thorac Surg 2001;71:827–31.

[37] Kalawski R, Deskur E, Bugajski P, et al. Stimulation of neutrophil integrin expression during coronary artery bypass grafting: comparison of crystalloid and blood cardioplegia solutions. J Thorac Cardiovasc Surg 2000;119(6):1270–7.

[38] Christakis GT, Weisel RD, Fremes SE, et al. Coronary artery bypass surgery in patients with poor ventricular function. J Thorac Cardiovasc Surg 1992; 103:1083–92.

[39] Elveres OP, Korvald C, Ytrebo LM, et al. Myocardial metabolism and efficiency after warm continuous blood cardioplegia. Ann Thorac Surg 2000;69: 1799–805.

[40] The Warm Heart Investigators. Randomised trial of normothermic versus hypothermic coronary bypass surgery. Lancet 1994;343(8897):559–63.

[41] Fremes SF, Tamaritz MG, Abramov D, et al. Late results of the Warm Heart Trial. The influence of non fatal cardiac events on late survival. Circulation 2000;102(19 Suppl 3):111:339–45.

[42] Mallidi HR, Sever J, Tamariz M, et al. The short-term and long-term effects of warm or tepid cardioplegia. J Thorac Cardiovasc Surg 2003;125(3): 711–20.

[43] Teoh KH, Christakis GT, Weisel RD, et al. Accelerated myocardial metabolic recovery with terminal warm blood cardioplegia (hot shot). J Thorac Cardiovasc Surg 1986;91:888–95.

[44] Menasché P, Subayi JB, Veyssié L, et al. Efficacy of coronary sinus cardioplegia in patients with complete coronary artery occlusions. Ann Thorac Surg 1991;51:418–23.

[45] Kaul TK, Agnihotri AK, Fields BL, et al. Coronary artery bypass grafting in patients with an ejection fraction of twenty percent or less. J Thorac Cardiovasc Surg 1996;111(5):1001–12.

[46] Borger MA, Rao V, Weisel RD, et al. Reoperative coronary bypass surgery: effect of patent grafts and retrograde cardioplegia. J Thorac Cardiovasc Surg 2001;121(1):83–90.

[47] The Warm Heart Investigators. Normothermic versus hypothermic cardiac surgery: a randomized trial in 1732 coronary bypass patients. Lancet 1994;343: 559–63.

[48] Cohen G, Borger MA, Weisel RD, et al. Intraoperative myocardial protection: current trends and future perspectives. Ann Thorac Surg 1999;68(5): 1995–2001.

[49] Lazar HL, Buckberg GD, Manganaro AJ, et al. Myocardial energy replenishment and reversal of ischemic damage by substrate enhancement of secondary blood cardioplegia with amino acids during reperfusion. J Thorac Cardiovasc Surg 1980;80: 350–9.

[50] Ericsson AB, Takeshima S, Vaage J. Simultaneous antegrade and retrograde delivery of continuous warm blood cardioplegia after global ischemia. J Thorac Cardiovasc Surg 1998;115(3):716–22.

[51] Lazar HL, Buckberg GD, Foglia RP, et al. Detrimental effects of premature use of inotropic drugs to discontinue cardiopulmonary bypass. J Thorac Cardiovasc Surg 1981;82:18–25.

[52] Marra C, De Santo LS, Amarelli C, et al. Coronary artery bypass grafting in patients with severe left ventricular dysfunction: a prospective randomized study on the timing of perioperative intraaortic balloon pump support. Int J Artif Organs 2002;25: 141–6.

[53] Christenson JT, Simonet F, Badel P, et al. Optimal timing of preoperative intra-aortic balloon pump support in high-risk coronary patients. Ann Thorac Surg 1999;68:934–9.

[54] Powell WJ, Daggett WM, Magro AE, et al. Effects of intra-aortic balloon pump counterpulsation on cardiac performance, oxygen consumption and coronary blood flow in dogs. Circ Res 1970;26:753–5.

[55] Christenson JT, Cohen M, Ferguson JJ III, et al. Trends in intraaortic balloon counterpulsation complications and outcomes in cardiac surgery. Ann Thorac Surg 2002;74:1086–91.

[56] Lim CH, Son HS, Baek KJ, et al. Comparison of coronary artery blood flow and hemodynamic energy in a pulsatile pump versus a combined nonpulsatile pump and an intra-aortic balloon pump. ASAIO J 2006;52(5):595–7.

[57] Dietl CA, Berkheimer MD, Woods EL, et al. Efficacy and cost effectiveness of pre-operative intra-aortic balloon pump patients with ejection fraction of 0.25 or less. Ann Thorac Surg 1996;62:401–8.

[58] Baldwin RT, Slogoff S, Noon GP, et al. A model to predict survival at time of postcardiotomy intra aortic balloon pump insertion. Ann Thorac Surg 1993; 55:908–13.

[59] Christenson JT, Simonet F, Badel P, et al. The effect of preoperative intra-aortic balloon pump support in patients with coronary artery disease, poor left ventricular function (LVEF < 40%) and hypertensive LV hypertrophy. Thorac Cardiovasc Surg 1997;45(2): 60–4.

[60] Torchiana DF, Hirsch G, Buckley MJ, et al. Intra-aortic balloon pumping for cardiac support: trends in practice and outcome 1968–1995. J Thorac Cardiovasc Surg 1997;113(4):758–69.

[61] Ferguson JJ, Cohen M, Freedman RJ, et al. The current practice of intra-aortic balloon counterpulsation. Results from the Benchmark Registry. J Am Coll Cardiol 2001;38:1456–62.

[62] Christenson JT, Cohen M, Ferguson JJ, et al. Society of Thoracic Surgeons (USA) National Database. Trends in intra-aortic balloon counterpulsation complications and outcomes in cardiac surgery. Ann Thorac Surg 2002;74:1086–91.

[63] Busch T, Sirbu H, Zenker D, et al. Vascular complications related to intra-aortic counterpulsation: an analysis of a 10-year experience. Thoracic Cardiovascular Surgery 1997; 45:55–9.

[64] Ivanov J, Weisel RD, David TE, et al. Fifteen-year trends in risk severity and operative mortality in elderly patients undergoing coronary artery bypass graft surgery. Circulation 1998;97(7):673–80.

[65] Yau TM, Fedak PWM, Weisel RD, et al. Predictors of operative risk for coronary bypass operations in patients with left ventricular dysfunction. J Thorac Cardiovasc Surg 1999;118(6):1006–13.

[66] Wechsler AS. Coronary artery bypass grafting in patients with an ejection fraction of twenty percent or less. J Thorac Cardiovasc Surg 1996;111:998–1000.

[67] Gutfinger DE, Ott RA, Miller M, et al. Aggressive pre-operative use of intra-aortic balloon pump in elderly patients undergoing coronary artery bypass grafting. Ann Thorac Surg 1999;67:610–3.

[68] Baskett RJ, O'Connor GT, Hirsch GM, et al. A multi-center comparison of intra-aortic balloon pump in isolated coronary bypass graft surgery. Ann Thorac Surg 2003;76(6):1988–92.

[69] Holman W, Qing L, Kiefe C, et al. Prophylactic value of precision intra-aortic balloon pump: analysis of a statewide experience. J Thorac Cardiovasc Surg 2000;120:1112–9.

[70] Wessel DL, Adatia I, Giglia M, et al. Use of inhaled nitric oxide and acetylcholine in the evaluation of pulmonary hypertension and endothelial function

after cardiopulmonary bypass. Circulation 1993;88:
2128–38.

[71] Fullerton DA, McIntyre RC Jr. Inhaled nitric oxide:
therapeutic applications in cardiothoracic surgery.
Ann Thorac Surg 1996;61:1856–64.

[72] Fullerton DA, Jones SD, Jaggers J, et al. Effective
control of pulmonary vascular resistance with inhaled nitric oxide following cardiac operation.
J Thorac Cardiovasc 1996;111:753–63.

[73] Girard C, Lehot JJ, Pannetier JC, et al. Inhaled
nitric oxide after mitral valve replacement in patients
with chronic pulmonary hypertension. Anesthesiol-
ogy 1992;77:880–3.

[74] Fullerton DA, Jaggers J, Wollmering M, et al. Variable response to inhaled nitric oxide following cardiac surgery. Ann Thorac Surg 1997;63:1251–6.

[75] Fullerton DA, McIntyre RC Jr, Hahn AR, et al.
Dysfunction of cGMP-mediated pulmonary vasore-
laxation in endotoxin induced acute lung injury. Am
J Physiol 1995;268:L1029–35.

[76] Fullerton DA, Jaggers J, Piedalue F, et al. Effective
control of refractory pulmonary hypertension after
cardiac surgery. J Thorac Cardiovasc Surg 1997;
113:365–8.

[77] Argenziano M, Choudhri AF, Moazami N, et al.
Randomised double blind trial of inhaled nitric oxide in LVAD recipients with pulmonary hypertension. Ann Thorac Surg 1998;65:340–5.

[78] Kieler-Jenson N, Lundin S, Ricksten SE. Vasodilator therapy after heart transplantation: effects of inhaled nitric oxide, and intravenous prostacyclin,
prostaglandin E, and sodium nitroprusside. J Heart
Lung Transplant 1995;14:436–43.

[79] Aaronson KD, Patel H, Pagani FD. Patient selection for left ventricular assist device therapy. Ann
Thorac Surg 2003;75:S29–35.

[80] Taylor DO, Edwards LB, Bouck MM, et al. Registry
of The International Society for Heart and Lung
Transplantation: Twenty-third Official Adult Heart
Transplantation Report—2006. J Heart Lung
Transplant 2006;25:869–79.

[81] Oz MC, Goldstein DJ, Pepino P, et al. Screening
scale predicts patients successfully receiving long
term implantable left ventricular assist devices. Circulation 1995;92(Suppl II):II169–73.

[82] Entwistle JWC. Short and long term mechanical
ventricular assistance towards myocardial recovery.
Surg Clin North Am 2004;84:201–21.

[83] Samuel LE, Holmes EC, Thomas MP, et al. Management of acute cardiac failure with mechanical assist: experience with the ABIOMED BVS 5000. Ann
Thorac Surg 2001;71:S67–72.

[84] Jett GK. Postcardiotomy support with ventricular
assist devices; selection of recipients. Semin Thorac
Cardiovasc Surg 1994;6:136–9.

[85] Guyton RA, Schonberger J, Everts P, et al. Post cardiotomy shock: clinical evaluation of the BVS 5000
biventricular support system. Ann Thorac Surg
1993;56:346–56.

[86] Samuels LE, Kaufman MS, Thomas MP, et al. Pharmacologic criteria for ventricular assist device insertion: experience with the ABIOMED BVS 5000.
J Card Surg 1999;14:288–93.

[87] Farrar DJ. The Thoratec ventricular assist device: a par-
acorporeal pump for treating acute and chronic heart
failure. Semin Thorac Cardiovasc Surg 2000;12:243–50.

[88] Hetzer R, Potapov EV, Stiller B, et al. Improvement
in survival after mechanical circulatory support with
pneumatic pulsatile ventricular assist devices in pediatric patients. Ann Thorac Surg 2006;82(3):917–25.

[89] Arabia FA, Tsau PA, Smith RG, et al. Pediatric
bridge to heart transplantation: application of the
Berlin Heart, Medos and Thoratec ventricular assist
devices. J Heart Lung Transplant 2006;25(1):16–21.

[90] Frazier OH, Rose EA, McCarthy P, et al. Improved
mortality and rehabilitation of transplant candidates treated with a long-term implantable left ventricular assist system. Ann Thorac Surg 1995;222:
327–8.

[91] Jett GK. ABIOMED BVS 5000: experience and potential advantages. Ann Thorac Surg 1996;61:301–4.

[92] Hoy FBY, Mueller DK, Geiss DM, et al. Bridge to
recovery for postcardiotomy failure: is there still
a role for centrifugal pumps? Ann Thorac Surg
2000;70:1259–63.

[93] Pae WE Jr, Miller CA, Matthews Y, et al. Ventricular assist devices for postcardiotomy cardiogenic
shock. A combined registry experience. J Thorac
Cardiovasc Surg 1992;104(3):541–52.

[94] Golding LA, Crouch RD, Stewart RW, et al. Postcardiotomy centrifugal mechanical ventricular support. Ann Thorac Surg 1992;54(6):1059–63.

[95] Lee WA, Gillinov AM, Cameron DE, et al. Centrifugal ventricular assist device for support of the failing heart after cardiac surgery. Crit Care Med 1993;
21(8):1186–91.

[96] Imasaka K, Masuda M, Oishi T, et al. Mechanical
cardiac support system for patients with postcardiotomy cardiogenic shock: analysis of risk factors
for survival. Jpn J Thorac Cardiovasc Surg 2004;
52(4):163–8.

[97] DeRose JJ Jr, Umana JP, Argenziano M, et al. Improved results for postcardiotomy cardiogenic shock
with the use of implantable left ventricular assist devices. Ann Thorac Surg 1997;64(6):1757–62.

[98] Westaby S, Balacumaraswami L, Evans BJ, et al.
Elective transfer from cardiopulmonary bypass to
centrifugal blood pump support in very high-risk
cardiac surgery. J Thorac Cardiovasc Surg 2007;
133(2):577–8.

ELSEVIER
SAUNDERS

Heart Failure Clin 3 (2007) 181–210

HEART
FAILURE
CLINICS

Surgery for Myocardial Salvage in Acute Myocardial Infarction and Acute Coronary Syndromes

George M. Comas, MD*, Barry C. Esrig, MD, Mehmet C. Oz, MD

College of Physicians and Surgeons, Columbia University, New York, NY, USA

Acute myocardial infarction (AMI) and acute coronary syndrome are major causes of morbidity and mortality in the United States. Most recent statistics estimate that 1.375 million patients have a coronary attack per year with the annual incidence of AMI at 865,000. Total-mention mortality due to coronary heart disease is 653,000 per year, making coronary heart disease the largest killer of Americans (males and females). AMI is fatal in one third of cases, with 250,000 deaths per year occurring before the patient reaches the hospital [1,2]. Complications of AMI include cardiogenic shock, ruptured ventricular septum, ruptured free wall with tamponade, papillary muscle dysfunction with mitral regurgitation, pericarditis, and arrhythmia. The death rate from AMI has fallen by nearly 30% since the 1990s, with in-hospital mortality from AMI falling from 11.2% to 9.4% from 1900 to 1999 [3]. Improvements in mortality and morbidity over the past decade have been attributed to innovations in pharmacologic treatment, interventional cardiology, as well as techniques in bypass surgery and circulatory support [4]. Surgery has played a key role in addressing emergent catastrophes with resultant improvement in mortality and salvage of myocardium in the aftermath of AMI. Surgery has also been shown to reduce long-term morbidity from AMI as a result of emerging knowledge, new procedures, and technical advances. This article addresses the pathophysiology, the treatment options, and their rationale in the setting of life-threatening AMI and acute on chronic ischemia. Although biases may exist between cardiologists and surgeons, this review hopes to provide the reader with information that will shed light on the options that best suit the individual patient in a given set of circumstances.

Pathophysiology of acute ischemia

Pathophysiology

Occlusion of an infarct-related artery (IRA) can lead to ischemia directly or reduce collateral flow to already ischemic or vascularly compromised areas. Consequences include arrhythmia, hypotension, and high left ventricular (LV) end diastolic pressure. As a result of no flow or low flow, myocardial damage can develop rapidly as cellular death evolves. In the first minute, contractile dysfunction within the ischemic zone results from sarcomere deterioration. Active systolic shortening progresses to passive lengthening. Within 20 minutes of IRA occlusion, cardiac myocytes have depressed function and show the stigmata of myocardial stunning. As occlusion persists, damage becomes irreversible. After 40 minutes of ischemia, reperfusion is able to salvage only 60% to 70% of viable myocardium. This value falls to 10% at 3 hours of ischemia [5]. Animal models have shown a zone of widespread transmural necrosis at 6 hours of localized myocardial ischemia [6]. In humans, irreversible damage occurs at 4 to 6 hours of ischemia. Thus, success of myocardial salvage is a function of time.

After excitation–contraction decoupling occurs acutely in the minutes following AMI, prolonged systolic and diastolic dysfunction occurs [7]. Cell death proceeds by way of apoptosis (programmed cell death) or oncosis (cell swelling), depending on available energy levels. Apoptosis, the main

* Corresponding author. New York Presbyterian Hospital, Milstein Hospital Building, Room 7-435, 177 Fort Washington Avenue, New York, NY 10032.

E-mail address: gc2124@columbia.edu (G.M. Comas).

1551-7136/07/$ - see front matter © 2007 Elsevier Inc. All rights reserved.
doi:10.1016/j.hfc.2007.04.006

heartfailure.theclinics.com

cellular response to sublethal ischemia and reperfusion, requires sufficient cellular ATP [8,9]. Cardiomyocytes survive by metabolic adaptation and optimizing energy use [10]. Apoptosis may persist for up to 60 days after AMI as seen in postmortem analyses where IRA occlusion correlates with apoptosis in the peri-infarct region up to 2 months after AMI [11,12]. In murine models, even small levels of apoptosis can induce ventricular dilation [13]. In humans, microscopic apoptotic levels correlate with ventricular dysfunction, dilation, and heart failure symptoms in the post myocardial infarction (MI) period [14]. Paradoxically, apoptosis has been observed to increase in early reperfusion after brief ischemia. This is explained by calcium ion influx leading to intracellular deposition, membrane destabilization, and cell death. Others have shown that reperfusion increases apoptosis in irreversibly damaged cells yet increases the overall yield of salvageable cells [15].

Ischemic changes and cellular damage are mediated by inflammatory processes. Polymorphonuclear leukocyte infiltration, fibroblast proliferation, and collagen turnover lead to ventricular remodeling [16]. Cox-2 expression is upregulated in apoptotic myocardiocytes as well as in the myocardium after 12 hours of ischemia. C-reactive protein levels are increased after AMI and can be predictive of negative remodeling [17]. TNF-alpha, an inflammatory cytokine, is released and depresses cardiac function [18]. Mice transfected to overexpress TNF alpha have been shown to develop dilated cardiomyopathy [19]. The inflammatory infiltrate disappears by 8 weeks [20].

Permanent IRA occlusion leads to negative remodeling, which occurs progressively. Side-to-side slippage of myocytes, myocyte death, and infarct expansion initiate the process. To compensate, surviving myocytes hypertrophy in the border zones and unaffected myocardium becomes hyperkinetic. During the early postinfarct phase, necrosis spreads and the infarct area enlarges. Hypertrophy is initially a compensatory mechanism for the loss of viable contracting myocardium. However, as apoptosis leads to myocyte loss, inflammation and fibrosis cause increased collagen turnover, with synthesis ultimately outpacing degradation. Consequently, progressive dilation occurs months after AMI. Ventricular enlargement with wall thinning and poor function is the terminal stage. A scar is observed 2 to 4 weeks after AMI. This may be evidenced by wall thinning or abnormal wall thickness and may be observed as an akinetic or dyskinetic segment. Long-term remodeling with changes in fiber orientation and an increase in LV end systolic volume index (LVESVI) leads to congestive heart failure.

The extent of injury at border areas is variable. A peri-infarct ischemic zone consists of myocardium at risk of necrosis. Aggressive interventions such as percutaneous coronary intervention (PCI), the intra-aortic balloon pump (IABP), coronary artery bypass grafting (CABG), and ventricular assist devices (VAD) can salvage myocardium at risk and improve function, especially if ischemia is ongoing Tables 1 and 2.

Rationale for medical treatment

Supportive noninvasive measures can optimize cardiac status. Supplemental oxygen should be supplied to maintain oxygen saturation above 90%. Intubation and respiratory support with positive end-expiratory pressure may be required if respiratory function is diminished due to cardiogenic pulmonary edema [21]. Narcotic analgesia can alleviate pain and anxiety, thus reducing heart rate and myocardial oxygen demand.

Narcotics blunt the catecholamine surge and can reduce preload and afterload. Potential adverse side effects include hypotension and suppressed respiratory drive. Nitroglycerin can be used to achieve vasodilation, reduced preload, and improved collateral flow. However there is a risk of hypotension and ventilation-perfusion mismatch. Because arrhythmia is the most common complication of AMI, lidocaine or amiodarone can be used. Most importantly, beta blockers can decrease mortality after AMI by lowering

Table 1
Predictive factors of poor outcome after acute myocardial infarction

Anatomy	Site of lesion
	Size of myocardium at risk
	Poor collateral circulation
Physiology	Arrhythmia
	Low coronary perfusion pressure
	High myocardial O_2 consumption

Data from Lee DC, Oz MC, Weinberg AD, et al. Appropriate timing of surgical intervention after transmural acute myocardial infarction. J Thorac Cardiovasc Surg 2003;125:115–9.

Table 2
Predictive factors for development of transmural myocardial infarction

	Odds ratio	P value
Shock	6.2	<.0001
Renal failure	3.227	<.0001
Reoperation (2+)	3.8	.0001
Hepatic failure	3.11	.025
Reoperation (1)	3.024	<.0001
Hemodynamic instability	2.26	<.0001
OR 6h-23h	1.965	.001

Data from Lee DC, Oz MC, Weinberg AD, et al. Appropriate timing of surgical intervention after transmural acute myocardial infarction. J Thorac Cardiovasc Surg 2003;125:115–9.

metabolic demand and protecting against arrhythmia at the risk of hypotension and bradycardia. Heparin can block further thrombus propagation. With signs of cardiogenic shock, vasopressors and inotropes are indicated with judicious fluid management to keep pulmonary capillary wedge pressure 16 to 22 mmHg. Pressors such as dopamine and dobutamine can maintain perfusion pressure, although they risk increased afterload and increased myocardial oxygen demand. Intensive care monitoring with arterial line and pulmonary artery catheter are indicated depending on the degree of instability.

Rationale for reperfusion

Ischemia causes adenosine triphosphate (ATP) production to fall, intracellular calcium to rise, and amino acid precursors to diminish. Reperfusion reverses these deleterious changes. Reperfusion protects threatened myocardium, limits infarct size, and rescues hypoperfused border areas that can become arrhythmogenic foci. By augmenting coronary blood flow while decreasing myocardial O2 demand (with beta blockade), mortality reduction can be achieved. The "open-artery hypothesis" refers to the claim that myocardial salvage depends on reperfusion, by way of thrombolysis, PCI, or CABG. The basis of treatment for AMI is the restoration of IRA patency and the reestablishment of the flow of oxygen and substrates to threatened myocytes. Numerous studies have correlated timely reperfusion and IRA patency with myocardial salvage, improved cardiac performance, and improved outcomes. Positron emission tomographic studies as well as thallium imaging demonstrate that the quantity of viable myocardium after AMI in revascularized patients is correlated with survival [22].

Over two decades ago, Reimer and colleagues [23] showed that the extent of infarction varied with duration of coronary occlusion. Border areas of the infarct zone undergo hypoperfusion and are especially threatened in the setting of hypotension, pressure overload, and sudden ventricular distension. Timely opening of the IRA by thrombolysis or revascularization improves survival and reduces postinfarct complications such as sudden cardiac death (SCD), congestive heart failure (CHF), and reinfarction [24]. Studies of patients receiving PCI showed that spontaneous reperfusion before PCI have quicker recovery from myocardial stunning, less cardiogenic shock, smaller infarcts, and improved outcomes [25]. White and colleagues [26] studied patients after first AMI treated with early thrombolysis. All patients had coronary angiography 4 weeks after AMI. Multivariate analysis showed that patent IRA, area supplied by the IRA, and LV function correlated with prognosis and survival. The importance of maintained IRA patency was also demonstrated in the Thrombolysis and Angioplasty in Myocardial Infarction (TAMI) study group [27]. One arm followed 810 patients who had AMI treated with thrombolysis. Coronary angiography at 90 minutes and 7 days after reperfusion was performed. In-hospital mortality was 4.5% in patients who had both early and late patency, 11% who had early patency only, and 17% who had neither early nor late patency. The Survival and Ventricular Enlargement trial showed that in patients after AMI with ejection fraction (EF) less than 40%, a patent IRA was in independent predictor of decreased late mortality [28].

Early reperfusion is crucial. Half the deaths from AMI occur within 1 hour of symptom onset. The greatest risk of ventricular arrhythmia occurs within 4 hours of symptom onset [29]. Reperfusion after AMI has been shown to be of benefit especially if done within 12 hours. Most clinical trials show maximal benefits of reperfusion within 24 hours [30]. Numerous studies on thrombolysis showed that the best outcomes occurred when the intervention occurred within 1 hour of symptom onset [31]. Early reperfusion optimizes LV function, myocardial salvage, and, ultimately, survival [32,33]. The Late Assessment of Thrombolytic Efficacy study followed 5711 patients who presented 6 to 24 hours after AMI and given tissue plasminogen activator (TPA) or placebo [34]. Patients treated within 6 to 12 hours had lower mortality than patients treated after

12 hours. Based on these analyses, early thrombolysis and PCI are both the standard of care for AMI with ST elevation (patients presenting at risk to develop transmural MI). ACC/American Heart Association current guidelines indicate PCI is indicated as the first intervention in the treatment of ST-elevation myocardial infarction (STEMI) within 12 hours of symptom onset in capable facilities with a goal of medical contact to balloon time within 90 minutes.

Late reperfusion has been theorized to promote peri-infarct hemorrhage, edema, contraction band necrosis, and ultimately "myocardial stiffening." [35]. However, late reperfusion (24 hours after AMI onset) has been shown also to benefit myocardial function [36]. Although the window for myocardial salvage has closed, cardiac performance and survival are enhanced in several (nonrandomized) studies [37]. The broadening of the open-artery hypothesis is referred to as the "extended paradigm." Studies show that that late perfusion improves adverse ventricular remodeling and decreases arrhythmias by improving flow to the peri-infarct ischemic zone.

In the 2nd International Study of Infarct Survival, patients receiving intravenous streptokinase up to 24 hours after AMI had increased survival [38]. Pizzetti and colleagues [39] followed a small cohort of patients who had anterior infarct and occluded left anterior descending coronary artery who had percutaneous transluminal coronary angioplasty (PTCA) within 18 days. Sixteen patients who had successful PTCA had improved LV function over a 6-month follow-up compared with 11 patients who had unsuccessful PTCA and showed worsening LV function and LV dilation. Montalescot and colleagues [40] studied patients 6 weeks after AMI with IRA stenosis greater than 70% and showed that PTCA was able to augment segmental wall motion. Carlyle and colleagues found that late reperfusion lead to decreased collagen turnover and more favorable ventricular remodeling [41]. However, these supporting observational studies are small and limited by selection bias. No large randomized controlled trials demonstrate consistent benefit to late opening of the IRA, especially in asymptomatic patients. Thus, American Heart Association practice guidelines on PCI reserve late revascularization for patients after AMI to patients who have symptomatic ischemia or LV dysfunction attributable to the occluded IRA [42]. Randomized control trials are warranted to better define the time-dependent benefits of revascularization, especially in patients who do not have inducible ischemia and intermediate angiographic flow grade.

Reperfusion benefit mechanisms

Studies have attributed the benefits of late reperfusion to many causes, some independent of myocardial salvage [43]. Delayed patency of the IRA may reperfuse a "stuttering" infarct, limit infarct expansion, and reduce silent ischemia. By rescuing hibernating peri-infarct myocardium, apoptosis is averted and infarct healing is improved [36]. Late reperfusion has been shown to result in a thicker, stiffer myocardial scar by modulating replacement fibrosis. An open IRA allows for inflammatory cells to infiltrate ischemic myocardium and stimulate fibroblasts to repopulate and produce collagen. Macrophages then digest and scavenge necrotic debris and leave a more durable scar. Refilling the coronary vascular bed also provides a stiffer scaffold-like support for the peri-infarct zone [44]. A well-vascularized bed provides a supportive framework that may allow for thicker, more durable scars that are more tolerant of radial stress [45]. Patients who have patent IRA or good collateral flow have been observed to have less frequent LV aneurysm formation [46].

It is possible that late reperfusion may alter ventricular remodeling, limit ischemic ventricular dilation, and regularize autonomic nervous system function. However, preventing negative remodeling is not likely to be chiefly responsible for mortality benefit because the survival curve for patients who hvae late perfusion shows most benefit within 30 days after AMI and little thereafter [47]. Van der Werf [48] compared patients who had early versus late reperfusion and found that patients who had later reperfusion had less improvement in survival and more improvement in ejection fraction. Survival benefit of early versus late reperfusion may be obscured by the fact that early reperfusion (thrombolysis or PCI) may save some patients who have low EF that would otherwise not survive and be offered late reperfusion.

Late reperfusion may contribute most significantly by enhancing electrical stability. Arrhythmic events are a common occurrence after AMI. Infarcted myocardium provides a precarious substrate easily perturbed by electrical stimuli. Consequently, arrhythmia is a cause of death in 40% to 55% of SCDs in the post-AMI period, independent of LV function [49]. Reperfusion can mitigate the arrhythmic tendency of post-AMI myocardium. In a dog model, Culkins and colleagues [50] showed that dispersion of refractoriness and inducibility of ventricular tachyarrhythmias was increased in the infarct zone. Low-amplitude high-frequency late potentials often originate in the peri-infarct border zone and can be detected by signal-averaged electrocardiography. In a dog model of AMI, Arnold and colleagues [51] showed that spontaneous ventricular tachycardia decreased in the first 4 days after AMI in dogs that had an occluded IRA revascularized within 4 hours (ventricular tachycardia incidence 13% with patent IRA versus 25% in occluded IRA, $P = .01$). Nonrandomized human studies have shown normalization of these arrhythmic markers with reperfusion. One study by Gang and colleagues [52] showed that the incidence of late potentials are significantly less in patients reperfused after AMI. Signal-averaged electrocardiography in 106 patients after AMI treated with tissue-type plasminogen activator (tPA) showed late potentials in 6% of patients who had documented patent IRA versus 32% with occluded IRA ($P = .01$). Moreno and colleagues [53] also showed that QT dispersion, an indicator of ventricular repolarization variation, also decreased in response to successful thrombolysis. Vagal activity, as measured by baro reflex sensitivity, improved in patients who had open IRA in a series of 359 patient studies by Mortara and colleagues [54]. Increased vagal tone is protective against ventricular tachyarrythmias and SCD. Another study by Hermosillo and colleagues [55] showed that IRA patency correlated with increased heart rate variability, a marker of a robust autonomic nervous system. Kersschot and colleagues [56] examined 36 patients 4 weeks after first AMI and showed that 12% of reperfused patients had induced sustained ventricular tachycardia versus 74% of nonreperfused patients. Looking at arrhythmia free survival in patients 1 year after AMI, Hohnloser and colleagues [57] demonstrated that an occluded IRA was an independent predictor of post-AMI arrhythmia. Thus, with arrhythmia as a major source of morbidity and mortality after AMI, restoring IRA patency can improve survival independent of its salvage effect on myocardial viability.

Although the culprit occluded coronary artery may be reopened or the lesion may be bypassed, recovery made be hindered by a lack of microvascular reperfusion. Patency of the IRA has been shown to minimize the extent of the infarction zone and halt the "wave front" of cardiomyocyte death. But myocardial salvage can be limited by the lack of microvascular perfusion, noted as the "no-reflow" phenomenon [58]. Restitution of epicardial blood flow cannot guarantee perfusion at the myocardial level. Studies have demonstrated poor microvascular perfusion with myocardial contrast echocardiography (with intracoronary microbubble injection) despite angiographically verified IRA patency (thrombolysis in myocardial infarction [TIMI] grade 3 flow) [59]. Thus, optimized reperfusion indicates epicardial IRA patency as well as restored microvascular flow.

The most basic marker of reperfusion is early resolution of ST segment elevation or absence of Q waves on the electrocardiogram. ST resolution is a noninvasive and reliable predictor of mortality that enhances prognostic power when combined with angiographic patency. Early resolution within 30 to 60 minutes predicts smaller infarct size, recovery of cardiac function, and improved survival [60,61]. Complete resolution within 180 minutes after treatment closely reflects relief of ischemia and is a better prognostic indicator than TIMI 3 patency. Thus, continuous 12-lead ST monitoring is useful in thrombolysis to document real-time dynamic reperfusion at the epicardial and microvascular level, useful for risk stratification and to catch failed reperfusion [62].

Measurement of serum cardiac markers is another valid method of estimating myocyte necrosis. Creatine kinase and creatine kinase-MB fraction, myoglobin, troponin I and T released during infarction have peak values and release patterns correlate with infarct size and ventricular function [63,64]. Cumulative marker release (area under the curve) reflects overall cellular injury. Reperfusion success can be documented as rapid "washout" of cardiac markers. Levels of cardiac markers can predict hospital mortality independent from TIMI flow grades [65].

Microvascular perfusion can also be assessed by myocardial contrast echocardiography. This technique is employed during angiography by injecting sonicated contrast into the newly opened IRA. Perfusion of the infarct zone can be visualized echocardiographically. Myocardial contrast echocardiography has demonstrated that microvascular perfusion remains insufficient in 25% of patients who have TIMI grade 3 flow [61,66]. Alternatively, Tc 99 m sestamibi single photon emission is a technique that evaluates infarct size and myocardial salvage. It is best performed after AMI treatment [67]. Cardiac MRI is a technique that will likely play a larger role in assessing microvascular coronary flow, tissue perfusion, and ventricular function in the future [68].

Because epicardial patency may not capture reperfusion success at the microvascular level, the open artery hypothesis has been shifted "downstream" as part of the strategy to enhance myocardial salvage and surpass therapeutic limits. Adjunctive therapies may enhance microvascular perfusion and protect coronary microcirculation. Examples include platelet glycoprotein IIb/IIIa inhibitors, anti-inflammatories, and agents that protect against reperfusion injury. Glycoprotein IIb/IIIa inhibitors can protect against platelet/thrombi microemboli and enhance endothelial function. Studies combining glycoprotein IIb/IIIa inhibitors combined with thrombolysis or PCI have augmented microvascular flow, accelerated epicardial reperfusion, and improved outcomes in small trials. ST monitoring studies have shown that thrombolytics combined with glycoprotein IIb/IIIa inhibitors have led to quicker and more long-lasting myocardial reperfusion versus thrombolytics alone [69]. Other prospective agents include inhibitors of complement activation, antibodies to adhesion molecules, and pretreatment with adenosine (before PCI). All potentially may limit ischemia reperfusion damage and prevent no-reflow phenomena [70].

Impaired myocardium in acute and acute on chronic ischemia

Insufficient blood supply causes injury to the myocardium and can be manifested in three different ways. First, infarcted myocardium is myocardium that has not survived a persistent ischemic insult. Cells that have died are replaced with scar tissue. The tissue is nonviable (scarred) and beyond salvage.

Myocardial stunning is caused by reperfusion after an ischemic insult. The tissue is acutely dysfunctional, but viability is recoverable if reperfusion is sustained. There is no cell death. But, evanescent severe episodes (<20 minute) of coronary occlusion can cause severe injury [71]. Contractility (active shortening) is impaired even after blood supply is re-established because of metabolic derangement. Likely mechanisms include calcium overload, generation of oxygen radicals, and excitation–contraction decoupling due to sarcoplasmic reticulum dysfunction [72]. Consequently, there is diminished energy use, insensitivity of myofibrils to activation, and matrix collagen breakdown. Typically, stunned myocardium is located at the border of the infarcted areas and can be exacerbated by high oxygen demand, coronary spasm, or cardiopulmonary bypass. Sequelae include arrhythmias and heart failure.

Hibernating myocardium refers to myocytes in which metabolic demand exceeds supply. Contractility is hindered but the injury process can be reversed with reperfusion [73]. The presence of hibernating myocardium is likely in patients who have unstable angina. Carlson showed that hibernating myocardium occurred in 75% of patients who had unstable angina versus 28% of patients who had stable angina [74]. Identifying and rescuing hibernating myocardium with aggressive revascularization can improve cardiac performance. Hibernating myocardium is chronically hypoperfused and may inhabit the peri-infarct region. Cardiomyocytes adapt to the oxygen deprivation by metabolic down-regulation, ultrastructural alteration, and expression of fetal proteins. "De-differentiation" may by a pathway to avoid apoptosis [75]. Revascularization effectively restores peri-infarct contractility, reverses regional dysfunction, and recovers the viability of hibernating myocardium [76]. This may be one mechanism whereby late revascularization improves cardiac function.

Differentiating viable myocardium from impaired myocardium plays an important role in deciding when and how to pursue revascularization. Thallium perfusion scans track the redistribution of thallium as an identifier of reversible defects [77]. Positron emission tomography scans highlight the degree of viability by tracking radiolabeled glucose use [78]. Dobutamine echocardiogram can separate hibernating and stunned myocardium by examining wall motion as the heart is challenged with chronotropes and inotropes [79]. MRI with gadolinium is a developing modality that can visualize unfavorable interstitial changes early as well as detect wall motion abnormalities and make volume determinations [80].

While hibernating myocardium can best be rescued by revascularization, stunned myocardium can be approached pharmacologically. One avenue is to block the formation of oxygen free radicals. Allopurinol targets the xanthine oxidase hypoxanthine pathway to reduce the production of superoxide anion radicals. However, clinical benefits have been elusive [81]. Anti-inflammatories such as iloprost have worked in animal models but are ineffective as adjuncts in the TAMI trial [82]. Recombinant superoxide dismutase, which scavenges oxygen free radicals, can ameliorate stunning. Unfortunately, it is not practical therapeutically because benefit occurs only if given before the reperfusion injury [83]. Calcium channel blockers in some studies have been shown to enhance recovery from stunning when compared with nitrate therapy [84]. Inotropes target viable nonischemic myocytes and can assist ventricular function until recovery from stunning occurs. This benefit must be balanced against the risk of increased oxygen demand. Mechanical circulatory assist devices can provide temporary hemodynamic support. In summary, impaired myocardium can be categorized as infracted, hibernating, or stunned. Extensive infarcted myocardium in the absence of ongoing ischemia is best addressed by medical management, ventricular restoration, or eventual transplantation. Hibernating myocardium can be rescued by revascularization. Stunned myocardium must be supported with medical management or mechanical assistance (IABP or VAD) as necessary.

Methods for reperfusion

Thrombolysis

Thrombolysis is the simplest and least-invasive way to achieve reperfusion of acutely occluded coronary arteries by dissolving thrombus. Thrombolytics, given in 40% of patients after AMI, is the most common means of reperfusion [85]. Numerous multicenter trials showed that thrombolysis with streptokinase (SK) or tPA is safe and effective in treating early AMI [86]. The GISSI trial (Gruppo Italiano per lo studio della Streptochinasi nell'Infarto miocardio) showed SK decreases in-hospital mortality [87]. This megatrial showed that mortality decreased after thrombolytic therapy, with the most benefit occurring in patients treated within 3 hours. Mortality was decreased by 47% in patients treated within 1 hour [87]. The 2nd International Study of Infarct Survival trial demonstrated that the odds of vascular death at 5 weeks fell by 20% in patients receiving SK and aspirin 13 to 24 hours after symptom onset [38]. The TIMI andEuropean Cooperative Study Group were both randomized control trials that showed tPA improved outcome after AMI.

SK and tPA were compared directly in the Global Use of SK and TPA for Occluded Coronary Arteries trial, which showed that tPA improved coronary flow, ventricular function, and survival to a greater degree [31,88]. Eleven thousand, two hundred twenty-eight patients who

had early reperfusion resulting in patent IRA had significantly lower mortality ($P < .001$) independent of left ventricular ejection fraction improvement. This suggested that protective mechanisms other than myocardial salvage could be responsible. Mortality in patients who had patent IRA 3 to 6 days after AMI was 6.3% (tPA) versus 8.8% (SK) at 1 year [89]; 30-day mortality was lowest in the tPA-heparin (4.4%), although patency rates at 30 days were equivalent. The Global Use of SK and TPA for Occluded Coronary Arteries-1 trial also showed that survival directly related to elapsed time from symptom to treatment with ~1% increase in mortality per hour of delay. Global Use of SK and TPA for Occluded Coronary Arteries-1 confirmed that early complete restoration of antegrade epicardial flow improved survival. Further, angiographic verification of patency correlated with decreased mortality (Table 3) [90].

More recent trials show the IRA patency after thrombolysis is 50% to 85% with a stroke rate of less than 1%. The TIMI study categorized epicardial coronary artery flow into grades to codify reperfusion based on angiographic criteria: flow grade 0 to 1 (failed reperfusion), flow grade 2 to 3 (epicardial patency, successful reperfusion). Corrected TIMI frame count corrected TIMI frame count was also developed to describe dynamic distal coronary flow and gave an angiographic "blush" score as an indicator of restored microvascular flow [91]. Anderson and colleagues [92] performed a meta-analysis of five international thrombolysis trials and showed that TIMI grade 3 patency of the IRA improved survival. Mortality correlated with TIMI score: 8.8% TIMI 0/1, 7% TIMI 2, 3.7% TIMI 3. Long-term follow-up was performed in the Survival and Ventricular Enlargement study that evaluated patients who had previous AMI and evidence of heart failure. After follow-up (average 3.5 years), mortality was 24% in patients who had occluded IRA and 14% in patients who had patent IRA ($P < .001$). Evidence of patent IRA within 16 days of AMI correlated with increased survival and fewer heart

Table 3
Results of the GUSTO-1 trial

GUSTO-1	tPA-heparin	SK-heparin
90-minute IRA patency	54%	40%
Overall mortality	6.3%	7.4%
Stroke rate	7.2%	8.2%
Cerebral hemorrhage	0%	0.9%

failure symptoms [28]. Gaudron and colleagues analyzed the longer-term clinical course of 70 patients after AMI [93]. Forty-five percent had progressive cardiac remodeling that was associated with increased mortality. The only significant predictor of adverse remodeling was low TIMI flow grades in the IRA 3 to 5 weeks after the acute event.

Thus, thrombolysis is effective and simple logistically. Although early administration is essential, community hospitals can be equipped to provide this therapy. Yet even when TPA activator is given with aspirin and heparin, effective reperfusion is only achieved in two thirds of patients and TIMI 3 patency is only obtained in one half of patients. Reocclusion is noted in one third of patients by 3 months [94].

Percutaneous coronary intervention

Primary PCI according to many studies is the safest and most efficacious first-line treatment for AMI. PCI can be performed immediately (as MI evolving), delayed (after AMI but during hospitalization), or electively (after stress test and during subsequent hospitalization). Coronary angiography and subsequent PCI is capable of quickly identifying the IRA and restoring antegrade blood flow [31]. PCI is successful in more than 90% of patients. Compared with thrombolysis, PCI has higher patency (TIMI grade 3 flow), less reocclusion, less recurrent ischemia, less reinfarction, and less stroke, despite similar effects on ventricular function and possible myocardial salvage [95,96]. PCI is frequently able to access side branches. Innovative techniques include protection devices and thrombosuction to prevent distal embolization (no reflow). Stents have been shown to be effective and safe even at institutions lacking surgical facilities [97]. PCI with drug eluting stents is a rapidly developing field with potentially less restenosis, acute occlusion, and decreased incidence of emergent CABG. Drug eluting stents may have increased late thrombosis compared with bare metal stents. The requirement for antiplatelet therapy represents a logistical challenge should CABG be indicated during acute hospitalization. The decision of which stent to use in the emergent setting is evolving. Thus, where available, PCI is a preferred modality, although results from different hospitals have considerable variation (Table 4) [98–102].

Outcome data is supportive of the use of PCI as first-line therapy for AMI. Several studies and

Table 4
Percutaneous coronary intervention versus thrombolysis

Trial		Death %	Reinfarction %
TIMI [99]	T+A	5.2	6.4
	T	4.7	5.8
TAMI [100]	T+A	4.0	11.0
	T	1.0	13.0
ECSGS [101]	T+A	7.0	4.0
	T	3.0	7.0
TIMI-II [102]	T+A	7.7	5.6
	A	5.2	3.1

Abbreviations: T, thrombolysis; T+A, thrombolysis and angioplasty.

meta-analyses, such as Primary Angioplasty in MI (PAMI) Study Group, demonstrate PTCA improves survival compared with thrombolysis [103]. Brodie and colleagues [104] showed patients who had patent IRA after primary PTCA had favorable long-term 5-year outcome and improved LV function. PTCA is possible even for complete occlusion. Shepo and colleagues followed 2007 patients with total coronary occlusion 7 days after AMI [105]. Patients who had successful PTCA had significant long-term survival advantage over patients who had failed PTCA with outcomes comparable with those without complete occlusion. Late PCI has been shown to be helpful. The Total Occlusion Angioplasty STudy-Società Italiana di Cardiologia Invasiva study examined 376 patients who had total coronary occlusion over 30 days after AMI (50% presented after 90 days) were treated with PCI (96% had stents) [106]. At 1-year follow-up, patients who had successful recanalization had mortality of 1% versus 7% with unsuccessful recanalization ($P = .008$). The Treatment of Post Thrombolytic Stenoses study group showed no improvement with late PCI after AMI treated with thrombolysis if the patient had no inducible ischemia on stress test [107]. The TIMI-IIb study supported PTCA after thrombolysis if symptoms persisted or if there was inducible ischemia.

Studies supporting PCI use have been criticized for selection bias. Furthermore, widespread use of PCI is limited by the availability of an operational catheterization lab and specialized personnel. An optimally functioning and rapidly deployable cardiac catheterization lab requires sophisticated coordination and a dedicated staff [108]. This may not be economically possible for every community hospital. On the local level, efforts must be focused on early diagnosis of

STEMI, medical stabilization, risk stratification, and expeditious transport to a catheterization facility. Surgical facilities should be available to assist in management. Urgent workup and initiation of therapy is crucial. IABP may be required for hemodynamic stability [109]. Echocardiography is useful to assess LV function [110]. Patients who have multivessel disease may need further revascularization if symptoms persist or there is evidence of recurrent ischemia. Thallium scintigraphy can assess for restenosis or recurrent ischemia. Thus, thrombolysis and PCI can both be considered first-line interventions for AMI depending on the capabilities of the treatment location. A patient in cardiogenic shock would benefit from immediate PCI as opposed to stabilization then delayed thrombolysis. If first-line thrombolysis fails and ischemia is persistent, then emergent rescue PCI is warranted. If a patient improves after thrombolysis, yet recurrent symptoms or inducible ischemia is noted, elective PCI or surgery before hospital discharge is indicated.

Surgical intervention

Surgery plays an important role in the management of AMI, a role that has been changing over the past decades. Advances in anesthesia, operative technique, and cardiopulmonary bypass (CPB) have made surgery safer and more effective. Recent improvements in myocardial preservation, controlled reperfusion, and mechanical circulatory support have fortified the options offered by surgery. Increased LV function after subsequent VAD months later has been demonstrated [111]. Even if there is a large amount of myocardium that is not salvageable, these measures may reduce adverse events and prevent further decline in cardiac performance.

Early studies showed that surgical revascularization within 30 days of infarct led to higher morbidity and mortality [112]. Poor results were attributed to hemorrhage into the infarct causing expansion of the infarct region. Conservative medical management was preferred, with the exception of absolute surgical indications of mechanical complications such as papillary muscle rupture with subsequent mitral regurgitation, LV rupture, and ventral septal defect. In the 1980s, published mortality after surgical revascularization was less than 5%, and CABG was preferred by many over medical therapy for AMI [113]. However, critics claimed that these reports were limited because such studies were not randomized

and subject to selection bias [114]. After thrombolytics and PCI came to the forefront, multicenter randomized controlled trials focused on comparing their relative efficacy. Thus, randomized controlled trials have never properly characterized the benefits of CABG versus alternatives in AMI.

Frequently, CABG after AMI has had excellent results with logistics and close integration between community hospitals and tertiary care centers. Still, due to accessibility of facilities and rapidity of therapy, thrombolytics or PCI remain first-line options for AMI. CABG plays a critical auxiliary role in AMI strategy however. Failure of thrombolytics or PCI with acute occlusion may require emergent surgery. Postinfarct angina, persistent symptoms, or inducible ischemia after recovery from AMI also benefit from surgical revascularization.

Close to 5% of patients presenting with AMI receive CABG (emergent or urgent) as first-line treatment. Another 5% receive CABG before hospital discharge for failed PCI or for definitive management of multivessel disease or for repair of the mechanical complications of AMI [115]. The primary angioplasty in myocardial infarction-2 (PAMI-2) was the first comprehensive study of CABG's place in the AMI treatment strategy. This prospective controlled trial studied 1100 patients at 34 centers who had cardiac catheterization within 12 hours after onset of AMI. One hundred twenty patients had surgery before discharge (10.9%) of which 42.6% were elective and 57.4% were urgent or emergent [116]. Surgery was performed in 6.1% of the 982 patients who had primary PCI. Only 4 cases (0.4%) required surgery emergently for failed PCI. Fifty-three of 118 patients not having PCI (44.9%) required surgery. The subset of patients who underwent surgery was a high-risk group that had multiple comorbidities and negative risk factors (diabetes mellitus, triple vessel disease, older age, diffuse atherosclerosis, unstable angina). Remarkably, in-hospital mortality was only 2.9% in this population. In an analysis of this population, patients requiring surgery were older, more often diabetic, and more often had triple vessel disease. Internal mammary artery (IMA) grafts were used in 30% of patients. In-hospital mortality was 6.4% in patients undergoing urgent/emergent surgery, 2.0% in patients undergoing elective surgery, and 2.6% in patients not undergoing surgery. After multivariate analysis, early and late reinfarction rates were equivalent in patients undergoing and not undergoing cardiac surgery (Table 5).

Table 5
Indications for cardiac surgery before discharge

Indication	All (n = 120)	After primary PCI	Without primary PCI
Failed PCI	5	4	1 (elective PTCA 4 days after admission)
LM disease	26	9	17
Unfavorable anatomy for PTCA	62	31	31
Recurrent unstable angina	18	17	1
Mechanical Complications (MR, VSD)	6 (3,3)	3 (3,0)	3 (0,3)
Inducible V tach	1	1	0
Unspecified	2	2	0

Abbreviations: LM, left main artery; VSD, ventral septal defect.

Data from Stone GW, Brodie BR, Griffin JJ, et al. Role of cardiac surgery in the hospital phase management of patients treated with primary angioplasty for acute myocardial infarction. Am J Cardiol 2000; 85:1292–6.

Surgery required in the 6.1% of patients following primary PCI was indicated either for failed PCI, to address refractory recurrent ischemia, or for definitive revascularization not amenable to PCI (severe left main coronary artery disease, triple vessel disease). Surgery was first-line therapy in 5% of the studied population (4.5% of patients not having immediate PCI). Surgery as first-line therapy addresses hemodynamic collapse, mechanical complications, and management of ischemic ventricular tachycardia. In-hospital mortality was low in both groups (following PCI and first-line) justifying the use of surgery even in high-risk patients. Surprisingly, adjusted cumulative late survival free of reinfarction was similar in patients after emergent, urgent, or elective surgery. This implies that careful selection of high-risk patients (ischemic cardiomyopathy, triple vessel disease, recurrent ischemia) is an important factor in long-term outcomes in the subgroup of patients status post PCI. Left unanswered is the impact of the extent of pre-existing myocardial damage (ie, does the benefit of cardiac surgery depend to a significant degree on preoperative risk stratification of baseline factors?) In summary, reperfusion strategy should be judiciously tailored to clinical scenarios. An individualized approach reduces mortality, reinfarcton, hemorrhage, and stroke [117].

The PAMI-2 study examined the common scenario whereby patients are triaged to PCI, CABG, or thrombolysis based on clinical, hemodynamic, and anatomic considerations. This study demonstrates that although surgery was an infrequently used first-line therapy for AMI, it was crucial for successful therapy in 10% of the study population. Access to standby surgical options is a necessary complement to PCI. Although emergent surgery for failed PCI was only exercised in four patients (0.4%) in this large series, most often surgery was urgent or semielective. Surgery as an adjunct to PCI optimized outcome especially in high-risk patients who have extensive pre-existing myocardial damage.

Some limitations of the PAMI-2 study are apparent. IMA grafts were used in only 30% of patients. This suggests that in the emergent setting, the incentive to decrease operative time reduces the use of arterial conduits and may limit the extent of revascularization. Long-term outcomes may reflect this dynamic and may turn out worse when compared with patients who had delayed surgery [118]. The PAMI-2 study occurred before the widespread use of stents. New PCI options may rescue more patients from failed PCI who would otherwise need surgery [119]. Glycoprotein IIb-IIIa use is not included in the PAMI-2 study population, also potentially affecting outcomes and the need for surgery [120]. Patients in cardiogenic shock were not enrolled. Surgery plays a critical role in this population although mortality is still ~40% [121]. Postoperative blood transfusions were unusually high (~60%) and possibly a sequelae of urgent surgery in patients treated with heparin and aspirin. Perioperative MI rate of 5% was similar to patients who had elective surgery [122].

In summary CABG is a means of halting progression of ischemia and necrosis and minimizing infarct size. The advantages of CABG compared with PCI for AMI include:

1. Similar survival for CABG and PCI for AMI
2. Surgery is a definitive revascularization treatment with long-term IRA patency demonstrated in elective cases (90% IMA patency at 10 years)
3. Complete revascularization strategy with more vessels potentially treated (less accessible distal obstructions can be bypassed)

4. Reperfusion can be controlled to minimize ischemic injury and reperfusion injury

CABG as the first-line mode for immediate revascularization is stifled by data suggesting higher mortality for early CABG. There are no long-term randomized control trials comparing CABG versus PCI versus thrombolytics in the setting of AMI. Most of the trials are retrospective observational studies. Controls are usually medically treated patients, possibly an outdated group. Selection bias may exist in the surgical groups (Table 6) [123–127].

Controlled reperfusion is an essential part of the acute surgical reperfusion strategy. Controlled reperfusion can limit myocardial damage by using substrates that bind calcium, thus blocking its influx and intracellular deposition. This strategy also involves agents that stabilize the myocyte membrane and replete ATP stores, all part of a strategy to limit reperfusion injury. Reperfusion injury occurs as an adverse consequence of the return of oxygen and nutrients to metabolically deprived myocytes. As oxygen is resupplied, oxygen-free radicals are produced. Cells swell and may become permanently damaged. Epicardial reperfusion can paradoxically trigger damage in the microcirculation [128]. This injury is mediated by neutrophil infiltration, production of oxygen free radicals, activation of the complement system, and up-regulation of adhesion molecules, all hallmarks of the inflammatory process [129]. Arteriolar spasm, endothelial dysfunction and showered platelet microemboli can disrupt microvascular flow, a disruption that can persist even after the epicardial IRA is reopened [130]. Ischemic myocardial damage also obstructs tissue perfusion [131]. "No reflow" phenomenon may be a consequence of reperfusion injury. Microvascular dysfunction can lead to progressive LV dilation and poor LV contractility. Consequences of reperfusion injury include myocyte death, endothelial injury, stunned myocardium, and arrhythmia (Table 7).

In the setting of myocardial ischemia, CABG offers the advantage of controlled reperfusion and complete revascularization. Controlling the conditions of reperfusion and the composite of the perfusate may minimize reperfusion injury and maximize benefits if heart tissue is ischemic but not yet infarcted [132]. Surgical revascularization allows myocardium rested on bypass to be recovered with gradual controlled reperfusion using balanced chemically optimized perfusate (eg, Buckberg solution) [133].

Several experiments on ischemia and reperfusion in dogs undergoing proximal left anterior descending coronary artery ligation were performed by Buckberg in the 1980s [134]. If the heart was in a beating state after only 4 hours of ischemia, extensive reperfusion injury could be produced by normal blood reperfusion. Segmental shortening, LV transmural blood flow, and mitochondrial ultrastructure were measured. However, results showed that the structural and functional integrity of transmural myocardium could be preserved after 6 hours of ischemia by controlling the conditions and composition of reperfusion. Myocardial damage could be limited and improved immediate functional recovery regional contractile function could be realized after up to 6 hours of acute occlusion.

In addition, several other studies confirmed that reperfusate composition and method of delivery correlated with myocardial salvage, recovery of contractility, and reduction of interstitial edema [135]. Studies have shown the importance of duration of reperfusion and degree of reperfusion. Reperfusate can be altered to increase

Table 6
Risk factors for poor outcomes after surgery for acute myocardial infarction

Early CABG	CHF [123]
Urgent/emergent [124]	Decreased LV function, low EF
Age	Preop CPR
Renal insufficiency	Left main disease
Number of previous MI	Female
Hypotension [125]	Poor LV wall motion scor [126]
Reoperation	IABP preoperatively
Cardiogenic shock	TM AMI [127]

Table 7
Types of reperfusion injury

Lethal	Cell death secondary to reperfusion
Vascular	Progressive damage causes expanding zone of "no reflow" and deterioration of coronary flow reserve during phase of reperfusion
Reperfusion arrythmias	Mainly ventricular arrhythmia occurring after reperfusion
Stunned myocardium	Post ischemia ventricular dysfunction

Data from Kloner RA. Does reperfusion injury exist in humans? J Am Coll Card 1993;21:537.

oxygen delivery, mitigate acidosis, decrease edema, resupply substrates, and decrease calcium influx thus allowing myocytes to replenisch ATP. The Buckberg solution, administered during cardioplegia, is an erythrocyte-containing, basic hyperosmolar solution stocked with aspartate, glutamate, and calcium chelators (Table 8) [136].

In addition, myocardial oxygen consumption can be minimized by using warm induction and warm reperfusion. The heart can be arrested with cardioplegia thus minimizing demand but maintained normothermic so that enzymatic activity can replete ATP stores.

Controlled reperfusion is part of the strategy of salvaging myocardium in the acute setting. A patient who has an old infarct but new persistent ischemia that is life threatening must be approached in a way that maximizes myocardial salvage. Alternatively, a patient who has an old infarct and a new infarct that is in cardiogenic shock must be approached in a way that maximizes circulatory support.

Administration of the Buckberg solution is part of the overall strategy of controlled reperfusion, referred to as the "integrated technique." First, a bypass circuit is employed with LV decompression as needed. Antegrade cardioplegia with warm Buckberg solution is begun to resupply ATP levels. High K^+ cardioplegia is given for diastolic arrest. The Buckberg solution also delivers glutamate and aspartate, substrates of the Kreb cycle, which allows ATP generation to continue. The result is promotion of mitochondrial ATP production while minimizing ATP demand and use. Retrograde cardioplegia follows to promote sufficient cooling and arrest in ischemic areas. Retrograde cardioplegia is used to supply the capillary bed distal to the coronary stenoses. Uniform temperature is assessed. Following each distal anastomosis, cold cardioplegia is injected into each graft and aorta

at 200 mL/min for 1 minute. After the ultimate distal anastomosis, warm cardioplegia suffused with enriched blood is injected into each anastomosis and aorta at 150 mL/min for 2 minutes. The timing is orchestrated based on data that maximal myocardial oxygen consumption occurs in the first 1 to 3 minutes of ischemia. After the aorta cross-clamp is lifted, blood cardioplegia is infused into the graft supplying the infarct region at 50 mL/min for 18 minutes. Proximal vein grafts are subsequently anastomosed. Revascularization occurs in an order that addresses ischemic areas first. The reperfused empty heart is allowed to beat for 30 minutes before weaning from bypass to minimize metabolic demand. The use of the Buckberg solution preserves myocardium and improves outcomes. In one series of patients, overall mortality in patients who had acute coronary occlusion having surgical revascularization with controlled reperfusion using the Buckberg solution was 3.9% despite the high prevalence of multivessel disease and cardiogenic shock [137]. Mean postoperative EF was 50%. The time from AMI to surgical revascularization was on average 6 hours. This time limitation is supported by the previously cited experimental confirmation that mitochondrial ultrastructure function can be preserved in arrested vented myocardium up to 6 hours. This "integrated technique" is especially applicable to patients in cardiogenic shock, whereby average mortality was lowered to 9.1% in this series (Table 9).

This strategy is one feature unique to surgical revascularization. Although PCI and thrombolytics can achieve reperfusion, they cannot control it. Although the revascularization technique may not make a difference in the normal patient, the integrated technique is helpful in the actively ischemic patient. In this population, superior results are achieved with warm substrate enriched blood cardioplegia infused before cross-clamp

Table 8
Components of Buckberg solution

Component	Concentration	Purpose
Blood	20–30% Hct	O₂ delivery
THAM trishydroxylmethylaminomethane	pH 7.5–7.6	Buffer acidosis
Osmolarity	350–400 mOsm	Decrease edema
Aspartate, glutamate	13 mmol/L each	Replenish substrates
CPD Citrate phosphate dextrose	0.15–0.25 mmol/L-Ca	Limit calcium
Glucose	>400 mg/dL	Hyperglycemia
KCl	8–10 mEq/L	Cardioplegia

Table 9
Reperfusion with Buckberg solution cardioplegic acute myocardial infarction

		Deaths, N	Deaths, %
Overall		6/156	3.9%
Subgroup	LAD occlusion	5/95	5.3%
	Triple vessel disease	0/66	0.0%
	Age > 70	1/22	4.5%
	Cardiogenic shock	6/66	9.1%

Abbreviation: LAD, left anterior descending coronary artery.

Data from Allen BS, Buckberg GD, Fontan FM, et al. Superiority of controlled surgical reperfusion versus percutaneous transluminal coronary angioplasty in acute coronary occlusion. J Thorac Cardiovasc Surg 1993;105:864.

release followed by antegrade and retrograde cold blood cardioplegia. These methods may reduce reperfusion injury, limit infarct size, and maximize myocardial protection [138].

Aside from controlled reperfusion, many advances at different levels of care have maximized myocardial protection and sustained reperfusion with surgical revascularization. Beginning with improved anesthetic techniques and monitoring, preparation must be made to rapidly go on bypass in the event of extreme hypotension or cardiac arrest during induction. Transesophageal echocardiogram (TEE) monitoring occurs throughout.

The integrated technique described by Buckberg [139] using warm induction and warm controlled reperfusion aids in optimizing myocardial salvage. Intraoperatively, ventricular unloading affords myocardial protection by lessening wall tension and oxygen demand. Myocardial uptake has been studied in various states of myocardial workload. As expected, myocardial oxygen consumption is reduced with cardioplegia. Of note, dyskinetic muscle has high energy requirements: five times more than cardioplegia and half that of beating working heart (O2 demand 8–10 cc/ 100 g/min). Energy demands are best counteracted by ventricular decompression because energy consumption can be decreased by 60% with ventricular unloading. Beyond venting, diastolic arrest can further decrease basal oxygen demand by 30%. Cooling only removes the last 10% of cardiac oxygen demand.

Early CPB for systemic perfusion is the most urgent means to decrease myocardial oxygen demand. Coronary salvage catheters across stenotic lesions can remain until aortic cross-clamp,

if the IRA cannot be opened. Antegrade and retrograde catheters permit rapid cardioplegia before cross-clamp, and can maximally protect threatened myocardium. The Buckberg solution, as described previously, is used with warm induction to replenish ATP supplies. Ischemic myocardium is grafted first so that cardioplegia can reach the threatened region expeditiously. Before the aortic cross-clamp is removed, proximal anastomoses are completed so that reperfusion commences.

Postoperatively, the complication rate is higher in patients who have preoperative cardiogenic shock versus patients who do not have preoperative cardiogenic shock, 47% versus 13% [140]. Survival rates correlate with postoperative EF and LV size [141].

Other approaches to surgical revascularization include off-pump CABG. Off-pump coronary bypass graft (OPCAB) uses devices to achieve regional stabilization and thus avoids CPB, potential myocardial ischemia, cardioplegia, and hypothermia. Studies have shown that OPCAB has lower mortality, less blood transfusions, lower troponin levels, less time on mechanical ventilation, and shorter hospital stays [142]. Troponin levels and other inflammatory markers are also reduced [143,144]. Magee and colleagues [145] reviewed a large series of patients having CABG-CPB (6466) and OPCAB (1983). Using risk stratification and propensity analysis in an attempt to eliminate selection bias, CPB was associated with an independent increased risk of mortality (odds ratio 1.9). The rate of stroke in beating on-pump coronary artery bypass graft (ONCAB) and arrested ONCAB are the same. On the other hand, OPCAB may lead to incomplete revascularization, although this disadvantage may be outweighed by the advantages of OPCAB [146]. Currently, OPCAB accounts for 22% of isolated CABG procedures and is technically challenging because of target vessel exposure and cardiac shift. Long-term graft patency has yet to be proven equal to ONCAB.

Another advance in the approach to bypass grafting is right heart–assisted CABG. Right heart–assisted CABG is an alternative that avoids the adverse hemodynamic effects of cardiac displacement in OPCAB (mainly caused by right-heart compression) [147]. Here, an extracorporal bypass circuit is employed without an oxygenator. One study examined 4733 patients who had CABG and compared selective outcomes of four techniques: arrested ONCAB, beating ONCAB,

OPCAB, right heart–assisted CABG [148]. Consequently, mortality was higher in beating ONCAB (4.4%) versus arrested ONCAB (3.5%) and OPCAB (2.3%) (ANOVA $P = .04$). CPB with an arrested heart has morbidity associated with manipulation, cross-clamp, global ischemia, hypothermia, and hemodynamic variation. Although groups were not well matched in this study (patients who were more ill were more likely to have ONCAB), the study concludes that OPCAB and right heart–assisted CABG, as well as beating ONCAB, are safe for critically ill, unstable patients. As surgeons become more familiar with newer techniques, they may evolve into improved alternatives for high-risk patients (cardiogenic shock, recent AMI, or low EF) requiring surgical revascularization.

Surgical treatment for an index acute myocardial infarction

In the setting of an index AMI, a patient's condition can vary from STEMI, non ST elevation myocardial infarction (NSTEMI) (subendocardial), or cardiogenic shock. The approach begins with medical management (previously outlined) and then proper diagnosis. Surgery is an essential part of the treatment armamentarium in approaching all clinical scenarios. With a STEMI, PCI can identify and address the culprit vessel. With NSTEMI, PCI is less likely to identify a single culprit lesion, and CABG for complete revascularization may be exercised as an option with higher frequency.

Rationale for early revascularization

Theoretically, early revascularization (within 3 days) can limit infarct expansion, prevent adverse ventricular remodeling, and avert ventricular aneurysm rupture [149,150]. Ventricular remodeling develops after infarcted myocardium is reperfused. After acute infarction, myocyte death causes regional akinesis. Necrosis spreads from endocardium to epicardium. As fibrosis occurs, the wall segment begins to remodel. The surrounding myocardium alters its shape as the ventricle increases its volume. Fundamental architectural changes ensue as apical loop becomes more basal. The normal elliptical shape of the "helical heart" becomes more spherical, and systolic function deteriorates [151]. As the apical loop fiber angle orientation becomes more transverse, the 15% fiber shortening that once

produced a 60% ejection fraction now produces a 30% ejection fraction [152].

The long-term effects of ischemia and infarction that occur after AMI must be considered in the evaluation of initial treatments. Of these effects, LV dilation and remodeling are well documented as sequelae of AMI. Two thirds of cases of CHF are from coronary artery disease (CAD) with most these after MI [153]. Studies show that ventricular enlargement begins early and continues years after AMI. Pfeffer and colleagues [154] showed that progressive ventricular dilatation continues during the late convalescent phase after myocardial infarction. During 1 year of follow-up, the end-diastolic volume of the left ventricle increased by a mean of 21 mL ($P < .02$) in untreated patients, with a much greater increase in patients who had combined akinetic/dyskinetic wall area greater than 30%. Early LV dilatation is associated with adverse outcomes. Impairment of LV function, as measured by LVESV, is the major predictor of mortality after acute myocardial infarction. Relative risk for death after MI increases exponentially in relation to LVESV [155]. However, early reperfusion acutely leads to decreased LVESVI. White and colleagues [156] performed a double-blinded trial of SK to study the effect of thrombolysis on LV function after AMI. In patients who had first infarctions treated with SK, LVESV was decreased and LV EF was increased, 6 percentage points higher compared with placebo (59% versus 53%, $P < .005$). However, while early reperfusion protects the epicardial layer and stops wall attenuation and dyskinetic aneurysm formation, late LV dilation still occurs in 20% of reperfused patients who ultimately progress to CHF. Gaudron and colleagues showed that 14 of 70 patients developed progressive structural LV dilatation after first AMI while being followed for 3 years [157]. At first, this was compensatory, but later, the dilatation was noncompensatory and resulted in severe global LV dysfunction. In this group, depression of global ejection fraction likely resulted from impairment of function of initially normally contracting myocardium. The harms of ventricular dilatation were quantified by Yamaguchi and colleagues [158], who studied the postoperative course of patients who had ischemic cardiomyopathy (EF < 30%) who underwent CABG. Preoperative LV volume (LVESVI > 100 mL/m^2 versus LVESVI > 100 mL/m^2) correlated with 5-year survival (85% versus 54%, $P < .05$) and freedom from heart failure (85% versus

31%, $P < .05$). Migrino and colleagues [159] investigated the outcomes of the Global Use of SK and TPA for Occluded Coronary Arteries-1 trial and showed that even with early opening of the IRA (within 3 hours), a significant number of patients (17%) had elevated LV ESV (LVESVI > 40 mL/m²). Early dilatation after AMI even after successful reperfusion therapy strongly predicted early and late mortality.

The optimal timing of surgical revascularization after AMI is controversial. Historically, emergent CABG after AMI had higher mortality 5% to 30%, with especially poor prognosis in patients who had transmural (TM) infarcts [160,161]. However, early studies comparing CABG to medical treatment showed that surgical revascularization within 6 hours of symptom onset improved mortality over medically treated nonrevascularized patients. DeWood and colleagues [162] retrospectively studied 440 patients who had TM AMI. Starting CPB within 6 hours of AMI decreased short-term and long-term mortality and improved late event free survival. Hospital mortality for non-TM MI was 3.1% and for TM MI was 5.2%. Mortality for CABG within 6 hours was 3.8% versus 8.5% for CABG after 6 hours. However, the average patient age was 54 with mostly single and double vessel disease, exposing the study to criticism of selection bias. Main predictors of death were age, prior CABG, and shock.

Today's environment is different. The population is older, multivessel disease is prevalent, and safe alternatives such as thrombolysis and PTCA exist. The capabilities of PCI are improving. A recent study of the New York State cardiac surgery registry investigated the effect of timing in CABG after TM AMI with the goal of delineating the optimal timing in this population as part of a strategy to improve outcome after AMI. This was a retrospective multicenter analysis of 32,099 patients after CABG after TM AMI from 1991 to 1996 by 179 surgeons at 33 hospitals in New York State [163]. The average age was 65 with EF 46%. Overall mortality CABG after TM AMI was 3.3%. Mortality decreased as time between the MI and surgery increased (Table 10).

Multivariate analysis of 43 risks factors showed revascularization within 3 days of TM AMI was an independent predictor of mortality. Day 3 was a point of inflection between the steep rise of mortality after early surgical intervention and the lower mortality later. After 3 days, mortality rapidly approached baseline. Although the risk does not return to baseline until day 7, there is no trend to statistical significance of added risk from day 3 to day 7. The conclusion was that aside from absolute indications for emergency surgical procedure (ie, persistent ischemia, mechanical complications), a 3-day waiting period should be considered to allow this high-risk period to subside. The initial 3-day window is a period of heightened systemic inflammatory response with precipitously high C-reactive protein [164]. Limitations of this study include lack of uniformity among surgeons, institutions, myocardial protection protocols, surgical techniques, CPB methods and duration, and anesthesia (Table 11).

This study corroborates the current ACC/American Heart Association guidelines of rescue PCI as primary treatment for AMI. Waiting beyond the dangerous peri-infarct period has demonstrated survival benefit. From this study, patients who had TM and non-TM AMI showed different trends in mortality over the observed time course. Mortality in the non-TM group peaked at 6 hours then declined dramatically [138]. Thus, CABG within 6 hours of non-TM AMI or within 3 days of TM AMI is associated with increased in-hospital mortality. However, patients undergoing early operation likely were more unstable or in cardiogenic shock, thus artificially elevating the mortality.

Because early surgical vascularization after TM AMI increases risk, aggressive cardiac support including LVAD should be available. In some patients, waiting is justified to optimize surgical outcome. This requires careful patient selection, optimal timing of the operation, and

Table 10
Mortality after surgery for acute myocardial infarction

Overall mortality	14.2%	13.8%	7.9%	3.8%	2.9%	2.7%
Time of CABG after AMI	<6h	6h–1d	1–3d	4–7d	7–14d	>15d
Odds ratio	1.6	2	1.5			

Data from Lee DC, Oz MC, Weinberg AD, et al. Appropriate timing of surgical intervention after transmural acute myocardial infarction. J Thorac Cardiovasc Surg 2003;125:115–9.

Table 11
Mortality after surgery for transmural versus non-transmural myocardial infarction

Time interval	Mortality % TM MI	Mortality % Non TM MI
<6h	14	13
6-23h	14	6
1d-7d	5	4
>7d	3	3

Data from Lee DC, Oz MC, Weinberg AD, et al. Appropriate timing of surgical intervention after transmural acute myocardial infarction. J Thorac Cardiovasc Surg 2003;125:115–9.

preoperative support, possibly with IABP [165]. Along with the patient's comorbidities, the neurologic status and the prognosis for sustained quality of life are mitigating factors that influence the extent of surgical intervention

Surgical revascularization and sudden cardiac death

Most early deaths after AMI are due to arrhythmias. Beyond the acute setting, malignant ventricular arrhythmia is responsible for most cases of SCD in the years following AMI [166]. Consistently, studies have shown that surgical revascularization has an independent effect on the rates of sudden cardiac death. The Coronary Artery Surgery Study followed 13,476 nonrandomized patients who had heart failure over 5 years [167]. SCD occurred more in the medically treated patients than the surgically treated patients 4.9% versus 1.9% ($P < .001$). Survival was increased because of surgery in the patients who had triple vessel disease and heart failure. Sergeant and colleagues later followed 5880 patients who had CAD status post CABG for 10 years [168]. Patients treated with surgery had a freedom from SCD of 99.8%, 99%, and 97% at 1, 5, 10 years, respectively, after surgery. Thus, CABG is more protective from SCD than it is from MI or recurrent angina (Fig. 1).

Surgical revascularization in patients who have CAD with or without AMI may promote electrical stability by preventing ischemic myocardium from becoming an arrhythmogenic substrate. The CABG Patch trial analyzed 146 patients who had low EF after CABG with postoperative electrophysiologic studies. No survival benefit was attributable to implantable cardioverter-defibrillator over 4 years [169,170]. Every and colleagues [171] followed 265 patients who

had cardiac arrest and resuscitation, 32% of which had CABG surgery. Over a 10-year follow-up, CABG was an independent predictor of decreased likelihood of cardiac arrest (52% decrease risk of subsequent arrest). CABG surgery also was shown to improve abnormal signal averaged ECG parameters and enhanced resolution of late potentials, both markers of arrhythmogenic tendency [172].

Cardiogenic shock

Cardiogenic shock is a multiorgan disorder caused by LV dysfunction, which reduces cardiac output. Because of its complexity, there is no uniform definition in all studies. Clinical definitions predominate: systolic blood pressure less than 90 sustained, without hypovolemia, and with evidence of end organ hypoperfusion (cyanosis, cold extremities, oliguria, uop < 20/cc, CHF, mental status changes). Hemodynamic parameters are also relied on in Global Use of SK and TPA for Occluded Coronary Arteries-1 and SHOCK (SHould we emergently revascularize Occluded Coronaries for cardiogenic shocK) trials (cardiac index < 2.2 L/min/m^2, pulmonary capillary wedge pressure > 14 mm Hg, surgical ventricular restoration > 2400 dyn sec/cm5 [173,174].

The extent of cardiogenic shock is proportional to the degree of myocardial damage [175]. A 40% loss of functional LV myocytes is the chief contributor of cardiogenic shock [176]. Cardiogenic shock may also be caused by mechanical complications: papillary muscle rupture, ventral septal defect, free wall rupture (<10%) [177]. Baseline pre-AMI EF and extent of collateralization, and size and location of IRA are important determinants [178].

Cardiogenic shock resulting from AMI has an incidence of 5% to 15%, a level that has remained stable over the years despite advances in medical therapy [179]. Cardiogenic shock more frequently occurs after Q-wave AMI than non–Q-wave MI [180]. Other risk factors for cardiogenic shock after AMI include age, female gender, history of DM or stroke, and recurrent AMI [181]. The Global Utilization of Streptokinase and Tissue Plasma Antigen Activator to Treat Occluded Arteries (GUSTO-1) trial found four predictors (age, hypotension, tachycardia, CHF) and reported that 50% of the cases of cardiogenic shock occurred with nonanterior AMI [182]. Cardiogenic shock is also documented in cases of right ventricle infarct [183]. One report described

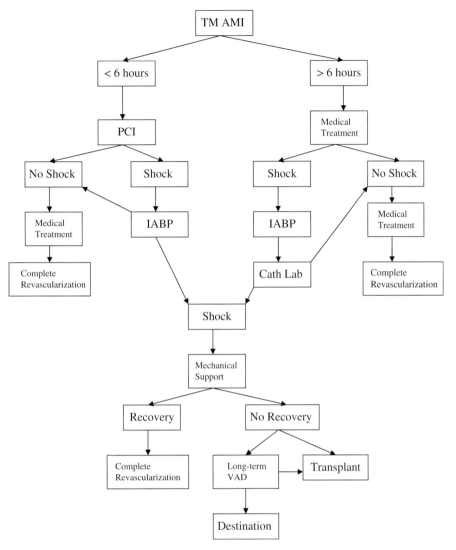

Fig. 1. Proposed algorithm.

cardiogenic shock after AMI having 71.7% in hospital mortality versus 12% mortality without shock [180]. Eighty percent of in-hospital mortality after AMI is attributable to cardiogenic shock [5]. Other reports list a 30-day mortality after cardiogenic shock from 47% to 77%, depending on treatment, ST elevation, and time interval from AMI to onset of shock (median time 6.2 hours) [184]. The median time from hospitalization for AMI to mechanical complications is 2.4 days.

In the case of cardiogenic shock, aggressive support and early intervention are critical. As previously outlined, medical management, including inotropic drugs, vasoconstrictors, and antiarrhythmic medication, should be instituted early. An integrated approach with anesthesia may be necessary, including early endotracheal intubation and monitoring with a pulmonary artery catheter. New PCI strategies to address total coronary occlusion, logistical improvements in hastening transfer to the cardiac catheterization lab, and development of glycoprotein IIbIIIa inhibitors have increased hospital survival, especially for high-risk patients [185]. Thrombolysis for patients who have cardiogenic shock has not improved survival [186]. However, as management practice is shifted from conservative to aggressive intervention, mortality in cardiogenic shock after AMI has declined.

Pumps such as the IABP are available to avert multiorgan system failure [187]. IABP is a temporizing adjunct useful in the early treatment of cardiogenic shock [188]. During systole, the balloon collapses and reduces afterload in the wake of this vacuum. In diastole, the balloon inflates and augments coronary artery perfusion by increasing intra-aortic pressure. This device reduces myocardial oxygen demand and enhances cardiac performance by decreasing afterload and improving coronary perfusion. Aortic counterpulsation is an important management strategy for acute coronary occlusion. It is most applicable in the scenario of cardiogenic shock [189]. IABP combined with early reperfusion has improved survival and recovery. Long-term follow-up has attributed use of aortic counterpulsation to less reocclusion and less recurrent ischemia with prolonged patency after reperfusion and without significantly increased vascular complications. Physiologic hemodynamic improvement is documented by less inotropic requirements.

Early aggressive intervention before multiorgan system failure and death from pump failure and arrhythmia is justified. Many studies confirm the importance of early resuscitation and revascularization. Hickman and colleagues [174] showed revascularization within 6 hours of diagnosis of cardiogenic shock improved survival especially in those aged less than 75 years. The GISSI I and II trials showed that mortality was 70% with thrombolysis [190]. PCI after cardiogenic shock improved survival to 40% to 66%, although most patients had an IABP [191].

The mortality of cardiogenic shock after AMI is reduced by 20% to 30% with prompt surgical therapy. Unfortunately, preoperative predictive factors are not fully evaluated to identify which patients are ideally suited for surgical therapy. The SHOCK trial showed that decreased time to early revascularization by PCI or CABG for patients who had cardogenic shock improved survival [192,193]. Emergency revascularization did not significantly decrease mortality at 30 days, but by 6 months, there was a significant survival benefit, compared with medical management. Early PCI or CABG within 6 hours of onset CARD shock had 1-year survival 46.7% versus 33.6% for late revascularization. SHOCK trial suggests that aggressive early revascularization may decrease mortality and improve outcome.

In the SHOCK trial, two thirds of patients who had cardiogenic shock after AMI had triple vessel disease. This suggests that completeness of revascularization may improve in-house survival for AMI complicated by cardiogenic shock. CABG may be more likely to achieve this goal than PCI. However, the SHOCK trial does not clearly address patient selection for PCI versus CABG or how outcomes relate to the completeness of revascularization because the numbers are small. PCI was the predominant approach and the groups were not randomized (CABG patients were more likely to have left main disease or triple vessel disease) [174].

Aside from the SHOCK trial, the benefit of CABG for cardiogenic shock is well documented [194]. DeWood and colleagues [195] showed that patients temporized with IABP then undergoing emergent CABG had mortality 25%, well below 80% of historical controls. In the GUSTO-1 registry, the 36 patients who had early CABG for AMI complicated by cardiogenic shock had 30-day mortality of 44% [196]. A meta-analysis of 26 studies reported that patients having CABG any time in hospital for AMI complicated by cardiogenic shock had hospital mortality 36%, although many of these studies may have suffered from selection bias. Mortality in patients surgically revascularized for cardiogenic shock due to nonmechanical causes ranges from 12% to 60%. Guyton and colleagues had 88% 3-year survival with surgical revascularization AMI and cardiogenic shock (Guyton and colleagues, Circulation 1987). Thus, the literature supports early surgery as valid alternative in the treatment of cardiogenic shock after AMI.

No demographic or hemodynamic factors were found while attempting to identify predictors of survival in patients who had cardiogenic shock undergoing CABG. Only two procedural factors were predictive: (1) longer time from AMI to procedure and (2) shorter cross-clamp time [197]. The longer time may be a confounder for a more stable shock patient.

Mechanical support

Considering the previously defined risk of surgical revascularization for TM AMI within 3 days onset, the preferred alternative is aggressive mechanical support for hemodynamic stability until elective CABG can be performed safely [124]. This delay can yield important clinical benefits if the case is nonemergent, especially for TM AMI. The VAD can rest stunned myocardium, protect against end organ injury, and support a failing heart as a bridge to ventricular recovery or transplant [198]. Ventricular unloading can provide support until recovery. Circulatory assistance can be vital to maintain hemodynamic stability. Delays can lead to permanent end organ injury. Mortality for cardiogenic shock after AMI can be as high as 80%. Patients in cardiogenic shock who undergo emergent CABG, who are unable to be weaned off bypass, and who require emergent LVAD insertion have poor outcomes. Better results are demonstrated in patients who have cardiogenic shock who receive a LVAD in a planned setting and undergo definitive surgical revascularization weeks later. Dang and colleagues [199] studied LVAD implantation in patients after anterior wall AMI and cardiogenic shock in 74 patients. Patients who underwent CABG before LVAD had higher early mortality, lower overall 6 month survival, and lower overall 12-month survival when compared with patients who underwent direct LVAD placement (39.10% versus 14.30%, 89.3% versus 54.4%, 82.1% versus 52.2%, $P < .05$). In addition, VAD placement has well-documented favorable results after postcardiotomy shock and intractable arrythmias. The benefits of mechanical support within the 6-hour to 24-hour timeframe extend to patients who had refractory cardiogenic shock from AMI as well. LVAD insertion remains an option in high-risk CABG patients (ie, patients who have persistent ischemia with poor EF after AMI or acute coronary syndrome).

Patients who are candidates for circulatory assistance can be put into two categories. First, patients who have stunned myocardium may need temporary ST support until recovery. Second, patients who have permanent myocardial damage may need support until eventual cardiac transplant (eg, young patients who have previously normal LV who have a large TM AMI). Short-term circulatory assistance may give enough support for the native heart to recuperate. However, if a patient who has CHF and a history of MI has an AMI with hemodynamic instability, a long-term device may be indicated as a bridge to transplant. Such patients can be supported for long periods. However, when devices are explanted, most redevelop CHF [111]. Future research is aimed at coordinating therapy with circulatory support to enhance return of cardiac function. Subgroups need to be identified where temporary LVAD after MI leads to full ventricular recovery.

Device use depends on specific needs of the recipient. Relevant selection criteria include:

1. Reversibility of cardiac injury, dependence on the device for functional recovery
2. Cause of cardiac dysfunction
3. Degree of right versus left dysfunction
4. Degree of circulatory support needed, expected duration of circulatory support
5. Patient age, size, comorbidities, patient candidacy for transplant
6. Location of myocardial injury
7. Contraindication to anticoagulation

There is an array of options for circulatory assistance. Short-term devices that can be inserted percutaneously include IABP and extra-corporeal membrane oxygenation. Minimally invasive, percutaneously inserted catheter pumps are also available. Vacuum-assisted pneumatic and electric pumps requiring sternotomy can be inserted for temporary univentricular or biventricular support. These pumps are more suited for stunned myocardium but can also be a bridge to transplant. The devices are inserted without removal of ventricular tissue and can be removed without cardiopulmonary bypass. When the pump is explanted, ventricular function is not constrained. The ideal scenario for these devices is short-term emergent support in the setting of cardiogenic shock. Alternatively, long-term pulsatile and rotary pumps can be implanted as destination therapy or as a bridge to transplant. These devices are most suited for patients in chronic heart failure. At Columbia, 80% of the overall LVAD population survives to receive a heart transplant. A more elaborate pump is a direct mechanical ventricular actuation device. This pump is an elliptical cup that surrounds both ventricles and sequentially compresses and relaxes like cardiac massage. Implantation requires thoracotomy. Cardiac output is augmented over prolonged periods [200].

Early experience with LVAD after AMI documented patient survival between 10% and 60%. One report describes a 60% discharge rate in patients treated with VAD after AMI [187]. However, emergent LVAD insertion after MI can have mortality up to 75% [201]. This was typically a patient who had preoperative AMI in postcardiotomy shock while weaning off CPB. These results discouraged widespread adoption of this modality. Later studies showed that ventricular decompression assisted myocardial recovery

[202]. By ventricular decompression, systemic re-perfusion, and hemodynamic support, infarct size is limited and myocardium is preserved [203]. Limiting MI extension improves ventricular function and may mitigate development of malignant arrhythmias [204].

Some centers delay LVAD implantation to allow for hemodynamic and end organ stabilization [205]. However, early mechanical support can improve survival after AMI and promote bridge to recovery or transplantation [199]. VAD can rest stunned myocardium while providing systemic perfusion and averting end organ injury. Preserved end organ function is an early predictor of survival after AMI [206]. Heart transplant before multiorgan system failure is essential for long-term success. Ventricular unloading can improve contractility in postischemic hearts. Although this population is high risk, survival is improved in patients status post-AMI receiving VADS. Circulatory support reduces cardiac work and oxygen demand when the ventricle is weakest and helps salvage border regions. The aforementioned studies further supported the argument behind early VAD insertion for circulatory support in the unstable patient after AMI with complete surgical revascularization at a later time.

One retrospective review of survival after LVAD insertion following AMI studied the influence of timing. Twenty-five patients were analyzed. The early group (n = 15) received the LVAD less than 2 weeks after AMI. The late group (n = 10) received the LVAD more than 2 weeks after AMI. The patients in the early group had lower perioperative mechanical right ventricle assistance but higher perioperative iNO use. Sixty-seven percent of the early group survived to transplant versus 60% in the late group. Seven percent of the early group survived to explant versus 0% of the late group. The study concluded that early identification and expeditious insertion of LVAD after AMI was favorable. This study showed that mortality in the early cohort (26%) was less than mortality in the late cohort (40%) (although $P > .05$). Overall survival to transplant or explant of 74% is comparable to other cohorts receiving similar devices, suggesting that recent AMI does not confer a survival disadvantage [207]. Thirty percent to 40% of patients in both early and late cohorts developed malignant ventricular arrhythmias. In other studies, post-MI ventricular tachyarrythmias had an incidence of 65%. In this series all eight patients who had perioperative ventricular fibrillation had electrical cardioversion and antiarrhythmic treatment and had no adverse consequences. Although many factors affect mortality post LVAD implantation after AMI, this study argues that early VAD after AMI can be safe and efficacious. A 2-week "recovery period" before LVAD insertion is unnecessary.

However, this was a retrospective study, not a prospective randomized controlled trial. Outcomes such as survival to transplantation are modulated by several external factors such as availability of transplant. Selection bias is a concern, although preoperative demographics and clinical features were comparable. In the setting of postcardiotomy shock and acute decompensation, IABP or temporary circulatory assist device can be used until the patient can be transferred to a tertiary care facility for long-term LVAD as destination therapy, bridge to transplant, or recovery.

In light of studies indicating higher mortality with early surgical revascularization, circulatory support may play a role in early hemodynamic stabilization until elective surgical revascularization is safe. The Columbia strategy is to insert short-term devices early because survival is only 7% if devices are implanted after cardiac arrest. Circulatory support is also useful as an aggressive rescue measure if surgical revascularization is complicated by pump failure.

One risk of pre-emptive use of mechanical support to delay CABG is overuse. Selection criteria and LVAD screening scale must be stringent. Because careful patient selection is critical for success in circulatory support, efforts have been made to design a preoperative VAD risk scale (Table 12).

Scores reflect end organ dysfunction (lung liver kidney) and operative limitations (right heart failure, bleeding). If the combined score is greater than 5, then survival is 30% and the patient benefits from measures to stabilize the patient before LVAD insertion. If the combined score is less

Table 12
Preoperative risk scale for LVAD placement

Criteria	Points
Urine output < 30 cc/h	3
Intubation	2
PT > 16 sec	2
CVP > 16 mm Hg	2
Reoperation	1

than 5, then the survival is 90% and patient qualifies for a short-term temporary LVAD [208].

Infection remains a risk associated with LVAD insertion. In the previous series, the most frequent cause of death in the early cohort was multi-organ system failure from overwhelming sepsis. Potential infectious sources may not be detected with early implantation. However, theoretically, prolonged hypoperfusion as a consequence of delayed reperfusion may also predispose LVAD recipients to infectious risks. Large prospective randomized controlled trials are needed to address this issue.

Right-sided circulatory failure (defined as requiring RVAD or iNO) is a common complication of AMI and was seen in one third of combined early and late cohorts of the aforementioned study. The use of iNO translated into less need for RVAD in this series [209]. This series further reinforces the notion that early use of therapeutic adjuncts for right heart failure is beneficial.

Even if heart transplant is not feasible as a therapeutic endpoint, LVAD as destination therapy has been validated. It may be considered in appropriate patients recovering from an acute insult, though this is not the patient population originally studied. As important as the criteria for circulatory support placement are the criteria for weaning circulatory support. LV recovery can be predicted by initial cardiac markers, EKG changes, and pre-event EF. If prognosis for recovery is poor, initial placement of a long-term device is justified. If recovery is expected, then the ventricle should be unloaded and decompressed for 3 to 5 days, given inotropic support (phosphodieterase inhibitors), and allowed to beat and eject. If TEE shows signs of improvement, the short-term device is removed in the operating room but kept on standby for 1 hour while the heart is monitored for signs of fatigue. If TEE shows no recovery by 1 week, explant is unlikely. At this juncture, the patient is upgraded to long-term device or support is discontinued if meaningful recovery is not achievable.

Surgical treatment for an acute event in chronically ischemic myocardium

STEMI and NSTEMI can occur in previously weakened or chronically ischemic heart tissue. PCI should be the first-line intervention with CABG to follow. In the previous sections, the authors outlined what also applies here, but in the acute on chronic setting, adjunctive procedures may be added.

To supplement the aforementioned measures, surgical ventricular restoration may be performed acutely in the setting of a LV aneurysm resulting from AMI. Large aneurysms can be resected with a patch of bovine pericardium sutured to the fibrotic edge of the inner ventricular wall (endocardium). Full-thickness myocardium is closed over the patch. Alternatively, the Dor procedure involves incising into the fibrotic scar of the aneurismal wall, excluding the scar with an endocardial suture and completing the repair with an endocardial patch. Excluding the scar restores elliptical shape to the ventricle and decreasing the LV volume. Some evidence supports improvement of systolic function [210]. Resection of small aneurysms is controversial and not routinely performed.

Surgical ventricular restoration can also be an adjunctive procedure in patients who have an old anterior infarct and a new lateral and inferior ischemia. Or, ventricular remodeling may be necessary for an anterior akinetic segment during a concomitant revascularization procedure. Consequences of ischemia include chamber enlargement and increased wall tension. White and colleagues [155] showed that increased LV volume was more predictive of survival that EF after AMI. LVESVI greater than 60 mL/m^2 had five times the mortality than normal volume after AMI (confirmed by the GUSTO-I trial) [159]. Systolic torsion is reduced as the dilated ventricle alters its shape from ellipse to sphere. Myofibril orientation moves away from the normal oblique axis to the transverse direction, providing the ventricle with less systolic function [211]. Thus correcting the LV geometry by way of surgical ventricular restoration improves EF. In the setting of ischemic cardiomyopathy, Yamaguchi and colleagues [212] described the long-term outlook after surgical revascularization as a function of LV volume. If LVESVI was greater than 100 mL/m^2, postsurgical outcomes were significantly worse. This provides the rationale for ventricular remodeling in association with surgical revascularization.

One study of survivors of AMI investigated how CHF was influenced by reconstructive endoventricular surgery. Early reperfusion can salvage myocardium and lead to akinetic wall. The RESTORE (Returning Torsion Original Radius Elliptical Shape to LV) study followed 1198 patients after AMI for 5 years who had surgical ventricular restoration, 95% of whom had CABG [213]. Surgical ventricular restoration improved ventricular function: EF increased from 29.6% to 39.9% with overall 5-year survival 68.6%. Various methods were used (direct closure or endocardial patch) with similar overall geometric objective. Excision of aneurysm with direct closure is no longer commonly performed because early reperfusion halts development of the dyskinetic thin walled ventricle [214]. Adverse remodeling develops around deeper scar and leads more often to an akinetic morphology [215].

MV repair, usually with ring annuloplasty, is often combined with surgical ventricular restoration (20% in the aforementioned series), usually in the subpopulation of extreme ventricular dilation. Patients who had MV repair added to CABG and surgical ventricular restoration have greater improvement in LVESVI. Surgical ventricular restoration is less helpful in remote segments such as when inferior and lateral wall are infarcted and asynergic [216].

Summary

Uncomplicated AMI can be managed in the community hospital by thrombolysis and medical management. Primary PCI, if available, may be more effective. Early, efficient resuscitation should begin, and expeditious transport to the cardiac catheterization lab and cardiac care unit are necessary to avoid delays in treatment. Surgical revascularization in a properly selected subset of these patients can yield good results if done in a delayed fashion. Thus, for most patients, acute surgical intervention is unnecessary.

However, patients who have mechanical complications, cardiogenic shock, or persistent ischemia benefit from early VAD or CABG. Acute complications of PCI or left main disease also require surgery. If there is no active ischemia and hemodynamics are recovering, surgery should be delayed until PA pressures fall. If surgery is attempted and there is difficulty weaning bypass despite inotropes and pressors (cardiac index <2 L/min/m^2, left filling pressures high, SvO2 $<$ 50%) insertion of a short-term VAD is indicated. However, evidence supports the conclusion that mechanical support is the best initial treatment of an unstable patient. The patient who has had an AMI but is not in shock has been demonstrated to not do well with surgery. However, the patient who has had an AMI and is in shock can be best treated with an IABP and VAD, if necessary, followed by delayed surgical revascularization if there is reversible ischemia.

Patients who have cardiogenic shock after AMI face high mortality (80% without surgery). Early reperfusion may play a critical role, although thrombolytics in this group are suboptimal. Early PCI is the first-line treatment in patients. Early CABG (in patients of age less than 75) is a viable option if pulmonary artery pressure less than 60/30 mm Hg and cardiac output greater than 3 L/min. Mechanical support becomes necessary if hemodynamics parameters are deteriorating and should pre-empt surgical revascularization. This approach can reduce the mortality of cardiogenic shock to 40% to 50%. In the emergent setting, a short-term VAD can provide circulatory support until the myocardium recovers and can be converted to long-term VAD if prolonged support is needed. A long-term LVAD should be placed if SvO2 is less than 50%. Surgical revascularization or VAD placement should be attempted in patients who are transplant candidates. If the patient is not a transplant candidate, then a conservative approach is favored because no safety net exists if CABG fails and mechanical support is required.

References

[1] Myerburg RJ, Castellanos A. Cardiac arrest and sudden cardiac death. In: Braunwald E, editor. Heart disease: a textbook of cardiovascular medicine. Philadelphia: WB Saunders; 1997. p. 742–79.

[2] Rosamond W, Flegal K, Friday G, et al. Heart disease and stroke statistics-2007 update. Circulation 2007;115: e69–171.

[3] Rogers WJ, Canto JG, Lambrew CT, et al. Temporal trends in the treatment of over 1.5 million patients with myocardial infarction in the US from 1990 through 1999: the National Registry of Myocardial Infarction 1, 2, and 3. J Am Coll Cardiol 2000;36:2056–63.

[4] Goldberg RJ, Gore JM, Alpert JS, et al. Cardiogenic shock after acute myocardial infarction. N Engl J Med 1991;325:1117–22.

[5] Jennings RB, Reimer KA. Factors involved in salvaging ischemic myocardium: effect of reperfusion of arterial blood. Circulation 1983;68(Suppl I): 1–25.

[6] Reimer KA, Jennings RB. The wavefront phenomenon of myocardial ischemic cell death, II: transmural progression of necrosis within the framework of ischemic bed size (myocardium at risk) and collateral flow. Lab Invest 1979;40: 633–44.

[7] Braunwald E, Kloner RA. The stunned myocardium: Prolonged, postischemic ventricular dysfunction. Circulation 1982;66:1146–9.

[8] Abbate A, Biondi-Zoccai GG, Baldi A. Pathophysiologic role of apoptosis in post-infarction left ventricular remodeling. J Cell Physiol 2002;193:145–53.

[9] Gottlieb RA, Burleson KO, Kloner RA, et al. Reperfusion injury induced apoptosis in rabbit cardiomyocytes. J Clin Invest 1994;94:1621–8.

[10] Bialik S, Geenen DL, Sasson IE, et al. Myocyte apoptosis during acute myocardial infarction in the mouse localizes to hypoxic regions but occurs independently of p53. J Clin Invest 1997;100:1363–72.

[11] Baldi A, Abbate A, Bussani R, et al. Apoptosis and post-infarction left ventricular remodeling. J Mol Cell Cardiol 2002;34:165–74.

[12] Abbate A, Bussani R, Biondi-Zoccai GGL, et al. Persistent infarct-related artery occlusion is associated with an increased myocardial apoptosis at postmortem examinations in humans late after an acute myocardial infarction. Circulation 2002;106: 1051–4.

[13] Wencker D, Chandra M, Nguyen K, et al. A mechanistic role for myocyte apoptosis in heart failure. J Clin Invest 2003;111:1497–504.

[14] Abbate A, Biondi-Zoccai GG, Bussani R, et al. Increased myocardial apoptosis in patients with unfavorable left ventricular remodeling and early symptomatic post-infarction heart failure. J Am Coll Cardiol 2003;41:753–60.

[15] Fliss H, Gattinger D. Apoptosis in ischemic and reperfused rat myocardium. Circ Res 1996;79:949–56.

[16] Hayakawa K, Takemura G, Kanoh M, et al. Inhibition of granulation tissue cell apoptosis during the subacute stage of myocardial infarction improves cardiac remodeling and dysfunction at chronic stage. Circulation 2003;108:104–9.

[17] Nifkardjam M, Mullner M, Schreiber W, et al. The association between C-reactive protein on admission and mortality in patients with acute myocardial infarction. J Intern Med 2000;247:341–5.

[18] Yokoyama T, Vaca L, Rossen RD, et al. Cellular basis for the negative inotropic effects of tumor necrosis factor-alpha in the adult mammalian heart. J Clin Invest 1993;92:2303–12.

[19] Bryant D, Becker L, Richardson J, et al. Cardiac failure in transgenic mice with myocardial expression of tumor necrosis factor-alpha. Circulation 1998;97:1375–81.

[20] Fishbein MC, Maclean D, Maroko PR. The histopathologic evolution of myocardial infarction. Chest 1978;73:843–9.

[21] Lee DC, Ting W, Oz MC. Myocardial revascularization after acute myocardial infarction. In: Cohn LH, Edmunds LH, editors. Cardiac surgery in the adult. 2nd edition. New York: McGraw-Hill; 2003. p. 639–58.

[22] Gioia G, Powers J, Heo J, et al. Prognostic values of rest-redistribution tomographic thallium-201

imaging in ischemic cardiomyopathy. Am J Cardiol 1995;75:759–62.

[23] Reimer KA, Lowe JE, Rasmussen MM, et al. The wavefront phenomenon of ischemic cell death. 1. Myocardial infarct size vs duration of coronary occlusion in dogs. Circulation 1977;56: 786–94.

[24] Welty FK, Mittleman MA, Lewis SM, et al. A patent infarct-related artery is associated with reduced long-term mortality after angioplasty for postinfarction ischemia and an ejection fraction < 50%. Circulation 1996;93:1496–501.

[25] Brodie BR, Stuckey TD, Hansen C, et al. Benefit of coronary reperfusion before intervention on outcomes after primary angioplasty for acute myocardial infarction. Am J Cardiol 2000;85:13–8.

[26] White HD, Cross DB, Elliott JM, et al. Long-term prognostic importance of patenct of the infarct-related coronary artery after thrombolytic therapy for acute myocardial infarction. Circulation 1994; 89:61–7.

[27] Ohman EM, Califf RM, Topal EJ, et al. Consequences of reocclusion after successful reperfusion therapy in acute myocardial infarction. TAMI Study Group. Circulation 1990;82:781–91.

[28] Lamas GA, Flaker GC, Mitchell G, et al. Effect of infarct artery patency on prognosis after acute myocardial infarction. The Survival and Ventricular Enlargement (SAVE) Investigators. Circulation 1995;92:1101–9.

[29] Marzilli M, Mariani M. Ischemia-reperfusion and microvascular dysfunction: implications for salvage of jeopardized myocardium and reduction of infarct size. Ital Heart J 2001;2(Suppl 3): 40S–2S.

[30] Sadanandan S, Hochman JS. Early reperfusion, late reperfusion, and the open artery hypothesis: an overview. Prog Cardiovasc Dis 2000;42: 397–404.

[31] The GUSTO Investigators. An international randomized trial comparing four thrombolytic strategies for acute myocardial infarction. N Engl J Med 1993;329:673–82.

[32] Sheehan FH, Doerr R, Schmidt WG, et al. Early recovery of left ventricular function after thrombolytic therapy for acute myocardial infarction: an important determinant of survival. J Am Coll Cardiol 1988;12:289–300.

[33] Cerqueiria MD, Maynard C, Ritchie JL, et al. Long-term survival in 618 patients from the Western Washington Streptokinase and Myocardial Infarction trials. J Am Coll Cardiol 1992; 20:1452–9.

[34] LATE study group. Late Assessment of Thrombolytic Efficacy study with alteplase 6-24 hours after onset of acute myocardial infarction. Lancet 1993;342:759–66.

[35] Pirzada FA, Weiner JM, Hood WB. Experimental myocardial infarction. 14. Accelerated myocardial

stiffening related to coronary reperfusion following ischemia. Chest 1978;74:190–5.

[36] Kim CB, Braunwald E. Potential benefits of late reperfusion of infarcted myocardium: the open artery hypothesis. Circulation 1993;88:2426–36.

[37] Galvani M, Ottani F, Ferrini D, et al. Patency of the infarct-related artery and left ventricular function as the major determinants of survival after Q-wave acute myocardial infarction. Am J Cardiol 1993;71:1–7.

[38] Second International Study of Infarct Survival (ISIS-2) Collaborative Group. Randomised trial of intravenous streptokinase, oral aspirin, both, or neither among 17,187 cases of suspected acute myocardial infarction: ISIS-2. Lancet 1988;2:349–60.

[39] Pizzetti G, Belotti G, Margonato A. Coronary recanalization by elective angioplasty prevents ventricular dilation after anterior myocardial infarction. J Am Coll Cardiol 1996;28:837–45.

[40] Montalescot G, Faraggi M, Drobinski G. Myocardial viability in patients with Q wave myocardial infarction and no residual ischemia. Circulation 1992;86:47–55.

[41] Carlyle WC, Jacobsen AW, Judd DL, et al. Delayed reperfusion alters matrix metalloproteinase activity and fibronectin mRNA expression in the infarct zone of the ligated rat heart. J Mol Cell Cardiol 1997;29:2451–63.

[42] Smith SC, Dove JT, Jacobs AK, et al. ACC/AHA guidelines for percutaneous coronary interventions. J Am Coll Cardiol 2001;37:2215–39.

[43] Fortin DF, Califf RM. Long-term survival from acute myocardial infarction: salutary effect of an open coronary vessel. Am J Med 1990;88(Suppl I): 9N–15N.

[44] Weisman HF, Healy B. Myocardial infarct expansion, infarct extension, and reinfarction; pathophysiologic concepts. Prog Cardiovasc Dis 1987; 30:73–110.

[45] Braunwald E. Myocardial reperfusion, limitation of infarct size, reduction of left ventricular dysfunction and improved survival: should the paradigm be expanded? Circulation 1989;79:441–4.

[46] Hirai T, Fujita M, Nakajima H, et al. Importance of collateral circulation for prevention of left ventricular aneurysm formation in acute myocardial infarction. Circulation 1989;79:791–6.

[47] Solomon A, Gersh B. The open artery hypothesis. Annu Rev Med 1998;49:63–76.

[48] Van de Werf F. Discrepancies between the effects of coronary reperfusion on survival and left ventricular function. Lancet 1989;1:1367–9.

[49] Raitt MH, Maynard C, Wagner G, et al. Relation between symptom duration before thrombolytic therapy and final infarct size. Circulation 1996;93: 48–53.

[50] Calkins H, Maughan WL, Weisman HF, et al. Effect of acute volume load on refractoriness and arrhythmia development in isolated, chronically infarcted canine hearts. Circulation 1989;79:687–97.

[51] Arnold JMO, Antman EM, Przyklenk K, et al. Differential effects of reperfusion on incidence of ventricular arrhythmias and recovery of ventricular function at 4 days following coronary occlusion. Am Heart J 1987;113:1055–65.

[52] Gang ES, Lew AS, Hong M, et al. Decreased incidence of ventricular late potentials after successful thrombolytic therapy for acute myocardial infarctions. N Engl J Med 1989;321:712–6.

[53] Moreno FL, Villanueva T, Karagounis LA. Reduction in QT interval dispersion by successful thrombolytic therapy in acute myocardial infarction. Circulation 1994;90:94–100.

[54] Mortara A, Specchia G, LeRovere MT, et al. Patency of infarct related artery: effect of restoration of anterograde flow on vagal reflexes. Circulation 1996;93:1114–22.

[55] Hermosillo AG, Dorado M, Casanova JM, et al. Influence of infarct-related artery patency on the indexes of parasympathetic activity and prevalence of late potentials in survivors of acute myocardial infarction. J Am Coll Cardiol 1993;22: 695–706.

[56] Kersschot IE, Brugada P, Ramentol M, et al. Effects of early reperfusion in acute myocardial infarctions on arrythmias induced by programmed stimulation: a prospective randomized study. J Am Coll Cardiol 1986;7:1234–42.

[57] Hohnloser SH, Franck P, Klingenheben T, et al. Open artery, late potentials, and other prognostic factors in patients after acute myocardial infarction in the thrombolytic era: a prospective trial. Circulation 1994;90:1747–56.

[58] DeWood MA, Spores J, Notske R, et al. Prevalence of total coronary occlusion during the early hours of transmural myocardial infarction. N Engl J Med 1980;303:897–902.

[59] Zeymer U, Schroder R, Neuhas KL. Patency, perfusion, and prognosis in patients with acute myocardial infarction. Herz 1999;24:421–9.

[60] Claeys MJ, Bosmans J, Veenstra L, et al. Determinants and prognostic implications of persistent ST-segment elevation after primary angioplasty for acute myocardial infarction: importance of microvascular reperfusion injury on clinical outcome. Circulation 1999;99:1972–7.

[61] Ito H, Tomooka T, Sakai N, et al. Lack of myocardial perfusion immediately after successful thrombolysis: a predictor of poor recovery of left ventricular function in acute myocardial infarction. Circulation 1992;85:1699–705.

[62] Klootwijk P, Langer A, Meij S, et al. Non-invasive prediction of reperfusion and coronary artery patency by continuous ST segment monitoring in the GUSTO-I trial. Eur Heart J 1996;17:689–98.

[63] Witteveen SA, Hemker HC, Hollaar L, et al. Quantitation of infarct size in man by means of plasma enzyme levels. Br Heart J 1975;37:795–803.

[64] Sobel BE, Bresnahan GF, Shell WE, et al. Estimation of infarct size in man and its relation to prognosis. Circulation 1972;46:640–8.

[65] Christenson RH, Vollmer RT, Ohman EM, et al. Relation of temporal creatine kinase MB release and outcome after thrombolytic therapy for acute myocardial infarction. Am J Cardiol 2000;85: 543–7.

[66] Ito H, Okamura A, Iwakura K, et al. Myocardial perfusion patterns related to thrombolysis in myocardial infarction perfusion grades after coronary angioplasty in patients with acute anterior wall myocardial infarction. Circulation 1996;93: 1993–9.

[67] Gibbons RJ, Miller TD, Christian TF. Infarct size measurement by single photon emission computed tomographic imaging with 99m-Tc-sestamibi: a measure of the efficacy of therapy in acute myocardial infarction. Circulation 2000;101:101–8.

[68] Wu KC, Zerhouni EA, Judd RM, et al. Prognostic significance of microvascular obstruction by magnetic resonance imaging in patients with acute myocardial infarction. Circulation 1998;97: 765–72.

[69] Maas AC, Green CL, Shah SA, et al. Incremental effects of anti-platelet, anti-thrombin, and fibrinolytic therapy on the speed and stability of ST-segment recovery after acute MI (abstr). J Am Coll Cardiol 2000;35(Suppl):372A.

[70] Marzilli M, Orsini E, Marraccini P, et al. Beneficial effects of intracoronary adenosine as an adjunct to primary angioplasty in acute myocardial infarction. Circulation 2000;101:2154–9.

[71] Bolli R. Mechanism of myocardial stunning. Circulation 1990;82:723–38.

[72] Marban E. Myocardial stunning and hibernation: the physiology behind the colloquialisms. Circulation 1991;83:681–8.

[73] Rahimtoola SH. The hibernating myocardium. Am Heart J 1989;117:211–21.

[74] Rahimtoola SH. The hibernating myocardium in ischemia and congestive heart failure. Eur Heart J 1993;14(Suppl A):22–6.

[75] Dispersyn GD, Mesotten L, Meuris B, et al. Dissociation of cardiomyocyte apoptosis and dedifferentiation in infarct border zones. Eur Heart J 2002;23: 849–57.

[76] Wijns W, Vatner SF, Camici PG. Hibernating myocardium. N Engl J Med 1998;339:173–81.

[77] Gibson RS, Watson DD, Taylor GJ, et al. Prospective assessment of regional myocardial perfusion before and after coronary revascularization surgery by quantitative thallium-201 scintigraphy. J Am Coll Cardiol 1983;1:804.

[78] Bergmann SR. Cardiac positron emission tomography. Semin Nucl Med 1998;28:320–40.

[79] Charney R, Schwinger ME, Chun J, et al. Dobutamine echocardiography and resting-redistribution thallium-201 scintigraphy predicts recovery of hibernating myocardium after coronary revascularization. Am Heart J 1994;128(5):864–9.

[80] Klein C, Nekolla SG, Bengel FM, et al. Assessment of myocardial viability with contrast-enhanced magnetic resonance imaging: comparison with positron emission tomography. Circulation 2002;105:162–7.

[81] Johnson WD, Kayser KL, Brenowitz JB, et al. A randomized controlled trial of allopurinol in coronary bypass surgery. Am Heart J 1991;121:20–4.

[82] Topol EJ, Ellis SH, Califf RM, et al. Combined tissue-type plasminogen activator and prostacyclin therapy for acute myocardial infarction. J Am Coll Cardiol 1989;14:877–84.

[83] Scott BD, Kerber RE. Clinical and experimental aspects of myocardial stunning. Prog Cardiovasc Dis 1992;35:61–7.

[84] Rinaldi CA, Linka AZ, Masaini ND, et al. Randomized, double-blind crossover study to investigate the effects of amlodipine and isosorbide mononitrate on the time course and severity of exercise-induced myocardial stunning. Circulation 1998;98:749–56.

[85] Hennekens CH, O'Donnell CJ, Ridker PM, et al. Current issues concerning thrombolytic therapy for acute myocardial infarction. J Am Coll Cardiol 1995;25(Suppl):18S–22S.

[86] Rentrop P, Blanke H, Karsch KR, et al. Selective intracoronary thrombolysis in acute myocardial infarction and unstable angina pectoris. Circulation 1981;63:307–17.

[87] Gruppo Italiano per lo Studio della Streptokinasi. Effectiveness of intravenous thrombolytic treatment in acute myocardial infarction. Lancet 1986; 1:397–402.

[88] The GUSTO Angiographic Investigators. The effects of tissue plasminogen activator, streptokinase, or both on coronary patency, ventricular function, and survival after acute myocardial infarction. N Engl J Med 1993;329:1615–22.

[89] Puma JA, Sketch MH, Thompson TD, et al. Support for the open artery hypothesis in survivors of acute myocardial infarction: analysis of 11,228 patients treated with thrombolytic therapy. Am J Cardiol 1999;83:482–7.

[90] Simes RJ, Topol EJ, Holmes DR, et al. Link between the angiographic substudy and mortality outcomes in a large randomized trial of myocardial reperfusion: importance of early and complete infarct artery reperfusion. Circulation 1995;91:1923–8.

[91] Gibson M, Cannon CP, Murphy SA, et al. Relationship of TIMI myocardial perfusion grade to mortality after administration of thrombolytic drugs. Circulation 1999;99:1945–50.

[92] Anderson JL, Karagounis LA, Califf RM. Meta-analysis of five reported studies on the relation of early coronary patency grades with mortality and

outcomes after acute myocardial infarction. Am J Cardiol 1996;78:1–8.

[93] Pfeffer MA, Braunwald E. Ventricular remodeling after myocardial infarction. Experimental observations and clinical implications. Circulation 1990;81: 1161–72.

[94] Wilcox R. Patency, perfusion, performance—the desirable triplets of combination thrombolytic therapy. Eur Heart J 2000;21:1495–7.

[95] Grines CL, Browne KF, Marco J, et al. A comparison of immediate angioplasty with thrombolytic therapy in acute myocardial infarction. N Engl J Med 1993;328:673–9.

[96] Natarajan MK, Mehta S, Yusuf S. Management of myocardial infarction: looking beyond efficacy. J Am Coll Cardiol 2000;2:380–1.

[97] Lindsay J, Hong MK, Pinnow EE, et al. Effects of endoluminal coronary stents on the frequency of coronary artery bypass grafting after unsuccessful percutaneous transluminal coronary revascularization. Am J Cardiol 1996;77:647–9.

[98] Christian TF, O'Keefe JH, DeWood MA, et al. Intercenter variability in outcome for patients treated with direct coronary angioplasty during acute myocardial infarction. Am Heart J 1998; 135(part 1):310–7.

[99] The TIMI Study Group. Comparison of invasive and conservative strategies after treatment with intravenous tissue plasminogen activator in acute myocardial infarction. N Engl J Med 1989;320: 618–27.

[100] Topol EJ, Califf RM, George BS, et al. A randomized trial of immediate versus delayed elective angioplasty after intravenous tissue plasminogen activator in acute myocardial infarction. N Engl J Med 1987;317:581–8.

[101] Simoons ML, Betriu A, Col J, et al. Thrombolysis with tissue plasminogen activator in acute myocardial infarction: no additional benefit from immediate percutaneous coronary angioplasty. Lancet 1988;1:197–203.

[102] Rogers WJ, Baim DS, Gore JM, et al. Comparison of immediate invasive, delayed invasive, and conservative strategies after tissue-type plasminogen activator: results of the thrombolysis in myocardial infarction (TIMI) phase II-a trial. Circulation 1990;81:1457–76.

[103] Keeley EC, Boura JA, Grines CL. Primary angioplasty versus intravenous thrombolytic therapy for acute myocardial infarction: a quantitative review of 23 randomised trials. Lancet 2003;361: 13–20.

[104] Brodie BR, Stuckey TD, Kissling G, et al. Importance of infarct-related artery patency for recovery of left ventricular function and late survival after primary angioplasty for acute myocardial infarction. J Am Coll Cardiol 1996;28:319–25.

[105] Suero JA, Marso SP, Jones PG, et al. Procedural outcomes and long-term survival among patients undergoing percutaneous coronary interventions of a chronic total occlusion in native coronary arteries: a 20 year experience. J Am Coll Cardiol 2001;38:409–14.

[106] Olivari Z, Rubartelli P, Piscione F, et al. Immediate results and one year clinical outcome after percutaneous coronary interventions in chronic total occlusions: Data from a multi-center, prospective, observational study (TOAST-GISE). J Am Coll Cardiol 2003;41:1672–8.

[107] Ellis SG, Mooney MR, George BS, et al. Randomized trial of late elective angioplasty versus conservative management for patients with residual stenoses after thrombolytic treatment of myocardial infarction. Treatment of Post-Thrombolytic Stenoses (TOPS) Study Group. Circulation 1992; 86:1400–6.

[108] Caputo RP, Ho KK, Stoler RC, et al. Effect of continuous quality improvement analysis on the delivery of primary percutaneous transluminal coronary angioplasty for acute myocardial infarction. Am J Cardiol 1997;79:1159–64.

[109] Stone GW, Marsalese D, Brodie BR, et al. A prospective, randomized evaluation of prophylactic intraaortic balloon counterpulsation in high risk patients with acute myocardial infarction treated with primary angioplasty. Second Primary Angioplasty in Myocardial Infarction (PAMI-II) Trial Investigators. J Am Coll Cardiol 1997;29:1459–67.

[110] Van de Werf F, Ardissino D, Betriu A, et al. Management of acute myocardial infarction in patients presenting with ST segment elevation. The Task Force on the Management of Acute Myocardial Infarction of the European Society of Cardiology. Eur Heart J 2003;24:28–66.

[111] Chen JM, DeRose JJ, Slater JP, et al. Improved survival rates support left ventricular assist device implantation early after myocardial infarction. J Am Coll Cardiol 1999;33:1903–8.

[112] Dawson JT, Hall RJ, Hallman GL, et al. Mortality in patients undergoing coronary artery bypass surgery after myocardial infarction. Am J Cardiol 1974;33:483–6.

[113] DeWood MA, Notske RN, Berg R. Medical and surgical management of early Q wave myocardial infarction, I: effects of surgical reperfusion on survival, recurrent myocardial infarction, sudden death and functional class at 10 or more years of follow-up. J Am Coll Cardiol 1989;14:78–90.

[114] Spencer FC. Emergency coronary bypass for acute infarction: an unproved clinical experiment. Circulation 1983;68(Suppl II):17–9.

[115] The Global Use of Strategies to Open Occluded Coronary Arteries in Acute Coronary Syndromes (GUSTO-IIb) Angioplasty Substudy Investigators. A clinical trial comparing primary coronary angioplasty with tissue plasminogen activator for acute myocardial infarction. N Engl J Med 1997;336: 1621–8.

[116] Stone GW, Brodie BR, Griffin JJ, et al. Role of cardiac surgery in the hospital phase management of patients treated with primary angioplasty for acute myocardial infarction. Am J Cardiol 2000;85:1292–6.

[117] Weaver WD, Simes RJ, Betriu A, et al. Comparison of primary coronary angioplasty and intravenous thrombolytic therapy for acute myocardial infarction. A quantitative review. JAMA 1997;278:2093–8.

[118] Campeau L, Lesperance J, Bourassa MG. Natural history of saphenous vein aortocoronary bypass grafts. Mod Concepts Cardiovasc Dis 1984;53:59–63.

[119] Stone GW, Brodie BR, Griffin JJ, et al. A prospective, multicenter study of the safety and feasibility of primary stenting in acute myocardial infarction: in-house and 30 day results of the PAMI Stent Pilot Trial. J Am Coll Cardiol 1998;31:23–30.

[120] Brener SJ, Barr LA, Burchenal JE, et al. Randomized, placebo-controlled trial of platelet glycoprotein IIb/IIIa blockade with primary angioplasty for acute myocardial infarction. ReoPro and Primary PTCA Organization and Randomized (RAPPORT) Trial. Circulation 1998;98:734–41.

[121] Stone GW. Primary PTCA in high risk patients with acute myocardial infarction. J Invasive Cardiol 1995;7:12F–21F.

[122] Coronary Artery Surgical Study (CASS) Principal Investigators and their associates. A randomized trial of coronary bypass. Circulation 1983;68:951–6.

[123] Kennedy JW, Ivey TD, Misbach G, et al. Coronary bypass graft surgery early after acute myocardial infarction. Circulation 1989;79(Suppl 1):I-73–8.

[124] Creswell LL, Rosenbloom M, Cox JL, et al. Intraaortic balloon counterpulsation: patterns of usage and outcome in cardiac surgical patients. Ann Thorac Surg 1992;54:11–20.

[125] Creswell LR, Moulton MJ, Cox JL, et al. Revascularization after acute myocardial infarction. Ann Thorac Surg 1995;60:19–26.

[126] Kouchokos NT, Murphy S, Philpott T, et al. Coronary artery bypass grafting for postinfarction angina pectoris. Circulation 1989;79(6 Pt 2):168–72.

[127] Stuart RS, Baumgartner WA, Soule L, et al. Predictors of perioperative mortality in patients with unstable postinfarction angina pectoris. Circulation 1988;78(3 Pt 2):1163–5.

[128] Kloner RA. Does reperfusion injury exist in humans? J Am Coll Cardiol 1993;21:537–45.

[129] Sheridan FM, Cole PG, Ramage D. Leukocyte adhesion to the coronary microvasculature during ischemia and reperfusion in an in vivo canine model. Circulation 1996;93:1784–7.

[130] Topol EJ, Yadav JS. Recognition of the importance of embolization in atherosclerotic vascular disease. Circulation 2000;101:570–80.

[131] Kloner RA, Rude RE, Carlson N, et al. Ultrastructural evidence of myocardial damage and myocardial cell injury after coronary artery occlusion: which comes first? Circulation 1980;62:945–52.

[132] Buckberg GD. Studies of controlled reperfusion after ischemia, I: when is cardiac muscle damaged irreversibly? J Thorac Cardiovasc Surg 1986;92:483–7.

[133] Allen BS, Buckberg GD, Fontan FM, et al. Superiority of controlled surgical reperfusion versus percutaneous transluminal coronary angioplasty in acute coronary occlusion. J Thorac Cardiovasc Surg 1993;105:879–84.

[134] Langer GA, Buckberg GD, Tillisch JH. Cardiac ischemia. Part II-reperfusion and treatment. West J Med 1987;147(1):54–61.

[135] Vinten-Johansen J, Buckberg GD, Okamoto F, et al. Studies of controlled reperfusion after ischemia, V: superiority of surgical versus medical reperfusion after regional ischemia. J Thorac Cardiovasc Surg 1986;92:525–34.

[136] Vinten-Johansen J, Rosenkranz ER, Buckberg GD, et al. Studies of controlled reperfusion after ischemia, VI: metabolic and histochemical benefits of regional blood cardiogenic reperfusion without cardiopulmonary bypass. J Thorac Cardiovasc Surg 1986;92:535–42.

[137] Allen BS, Okamoto F, Buckberg GD, et al. Studies of controlled reperfusion after ischemia, XII: effects of "duration" of reperfusate administration versus reperfusate "dose" on regional, functional, biochemical, and histological recovery. J Thorac Cardiovasc Surg 1986;92:594–604.

[138] Lee DC, Oz MC, Weinberg AD, et al. Optimal timing of revascularization: transmural versus nontransmural acute myocardial infarction. Ann Thorac Surg 2001;71:1198–204.

[139] Allen BS, Rosenkranz ER, Buckberg GD, et al. Studies of controlled reperfusion after ischemia, VII: high oxygen requirements of dyskinetic cardiac muscle. J Thorac Cardiovasc Surg 1986;92:543–52.

[140] Guyton RA, Arcidi JM, Langford DA, et al. Emergency coronary bypass for cardiogenic shock. Circulation 1987;76(Suppl V):22–7.

[141] Applebaum R, House R, Rademaker A, et al. Coronary artery bypass grafting within thirty days of acute myocardial infarction. J Thorac Cardiovasc Surg 1991;102:745–52.

[142] Demaria RG, Carrier M, Portier S, et al. Reduced mortality and strokes with off pump coronary artery bypass grafting surgery in octogenarians. Circulation 2002;106:5–10.

[143] Krejca M, Skiba J, Szmagala P, et al. Cardiac troponin T release during coronary surgery using intermittent cross-clamp with fibrillation, on-pump and off-pump beating heart. Eur J Cardiothorac Surg 1999;16:337–41.

[144] Caputo M, Yeatman M, Narayan P, et al. Effect of off-pump coronary surgery with right ventricular assist device on organ function and inflammatory

response: a randomized controlled trial. Ann Thorac Surg 2002;74:2088–95.

[145] Magee MJ, Jablonski KA, Stamou SC, et al. Elimination of cardiopulmonary bypass improves early survival for multivessel coronary artery bypass patients. Ann Thorac Surg 2002;73(4):1196–202.

[146] Sabik JF, Gillinov AM, Blackstone EH, et al. Does off-pump coronary surgery reduce morbidity and mortality? J Thorac Cardiovasc Surg 2002;124: 698–707.

[147] Mathison M, Edgerton JR, Horswell JL, et al. Analysis of hemodynamic changes during beating heart surgical procedures. Ann Thorac Surg 2000; 70:1355–60.

[148] Edgerton JR, Herbert MA, Jones KK, et al. On-pump beating heart surgery offers an alternative for unstable patients undergoing coronary artery bypass grafting. Heart Surg Forum 2004;7(1): E88–95.

[149] Isbir SC, Yildirim T, Akgun S, et al. Coronary artery bypass surgery in patients with severe left ventricular dysfunction. Int J Cardiol 2003;90: 309–16.

[150] Weiss JL, Marino N, Shapiro EP. Myocardial infarct expansion: recognition, significance, and pathology. Am J Cardiol 1991;68:35–40.

[151] Sallin EA. Fiber orientation and ejection in the human left ventricle. Biophys J 1969;9:954–64.

[152] Buckberg GD, Coghlan HC, Torrent-Guasp F. The structure and function of the helical heart and its buttress wrapping. Semin Thorac Cardiovasc Surg 2001;13(4):386–401.

[153] Gheorghiade M, Bonow RO. Chronic heart failure in the United States: a manifestation of coronary artery disease. Circulation 1998;97:282–9.

[154] Pfeffer MA, Lamas GA, Vaughan DE, et al. Effect of captopril on progressive ventricular dilatation after anterior myocardial infarction. N Engl J Med 1988;319(2):80–6.

[155] White HD, Norris RM, Brown MA, et al. Left ventricular end-systolic volume as the major determinant of survival after recovery from myocardial infarction. Circulation 1987;76(1):44–51.

[156] White HD, Norris RM, Brown MA, et al. Effect of intravenous streptokinase on left ventricular function and early survival after acute myocardial infarction. N Engl J Med 1987;317(14):850–5.

[157] Gaudron P, Eilles C, Kugler I, et al. Progressive left ventricular dysfunction and remodeling after myocardial infarction. Potential mechanisms and early predictors. Circulation 1993;87(3):755–63.

[158] Yamaguchi A, Ino T, Adachi H, et al. Left ventricular volume predicts postoperative course in patients with ischemic cardiomyopathy. Ann Thorac Surg 1998;65(2):434–8.

[159] Migrino RQ, Young JB, Ellis SG, et al. End-systolic volume index at 90 to 180 minutes into reperfusion therapy for acute myocardial infarction is a strong predictor of early and late mortality. The Global Utilization of Streptokinase and t-PA for Occluded Coronary Arteries (GUSTO)-I Angiographic Investigators. Circulation 1997;96(1): 116–21.

[160] Coleman WS, DeWood MA, Berg R, et al. Surgical intervention in acute myocardial infarction: an historical perspective. Semin Thorac Cardiovasc Surg 1995;7:176–83.

[161] Braxton JH, Hammond GL, Letson GV, et al. Optimal timing of coronary artery bypass graft surgery after acute myocardial infarction. Circulation 1995;92(Suppl 9):66–8.

[162] Dewood MA, Spores J, Berg R, et al. Acute myocardial infarction: a decade of experience with surgical reperfusion in 701 patients. Circulation 1983; 68(Suppl II):8–16.

[163] Lee DC, Oz MC, Weinberg AD, et al. Appropriate timing of surgical intervention after transmural acute myocardial infarction. J of Thorac Cardiovasc Surg 2003;125(1):115–20.

[164] Anzai T, Yoshikawa T, Shiraki H, et al. C-reactive protein as a predictor of infarct expansion and cardiac rupture after a first Q-wave acute myocardial infarction. Circulation 1997;96:778–84.

[165] Wasvary H, Shannon F, Bassett J, et al. Timing of coronary artery bypass grafting after acute myocardial infarction. Am Surg 1997;63:710–5.

[166] Bigger JT, Fleiss JL, Kleinger R, et al. The relationships between ventricular arrythmias, left ventricular dysfunction and mortality in the 2 years after myocardial infarction. Circulation 1984;69: 250–8.

[167] Holmes DR Jr, Davis KB, Mock MB, et al. The effect of medical and surgical treatment on subsequent sudden cardiac death in patients with coronary artery disease: a report from the Coronary Artery Surgery Study. Circulation 1986;73: 1254–63.

[168] Sergeant P, Lesaffre E, Flameng W, et al. The return of clinically evident ischemia after coronary artery bypass grafting. Eur J Cardiothorac Surg 1991;5:447–57.

[169] Bigger JT Jr. Prophylactic use of implanted cardiac defibrillators in patients at high risk of ventricular arrhythmias after coronary bypass graft surgery. Coronary Artery Bypass Graft (CABG) Patch Trial Investigators. N Engl J Med 1997.

[170] Bigger JT, Rottman JN, Whang W, et al. CABG surgery unlinked the arrhythmic substrate from arrhythmic outcomes in the CABG patch trial [abstract]. Circulation 1999;100(Suppl 1): 366–7.

[171] Every NR, Fahrenbruch CE, Hallstrom AP, et al. Influence of coronary bypass surgery on subsequent outcome of patients resuscitated from out of hospital cardiac arrest. J Am Coll Cardiol 1992;19:1435–9.

[172] Terada Y, Mitsui T, Matsushita S, et al. Influence of bypass grafting to the infarct artery on late

potentials in coronary operations. Ann Thorac Surg 1995;60:422–5.

[173] Alonso DR, Scheidt S, Post M, et al. Pathophysiology of cardiogenic shock: quantification of myocardial necrosis, clinical, pathological and electroophysiologic correlations. Circulation 1973;48:588–96.

[174] Hochman JS, Sleeper LA, Webb JG, et al. Early revascularization in acute myocardial infarction complicated by cardiogenic shock: SHOCK Investigators—should we emergently revascularize occluded coronaries for cardiogenic shock? N Engl J Med 1999;341:625–34.

[175] Gutovitz AL, Sobel BE, Roberts R. Progressive nature of myocardial injury in selected patients with cardiogenic shock. Am J Cardiol 1978;41:469–75.

[176] Wackers FJ, Lie KI, Becker AE, et al. Coronary artery disease in patients dying from cardiogenic shock or congestive heart failure in the setting of acute myocardial infarction. Br Heart J 1976;38:906–10.

[177] Hochman JS, Boland J, Sleeper LA, et al. Current spectrum of cardiogenic shock and effect of early revascularization on mortality: results of an International Registry—SHOCK Registry Investigators. Circulation 1995;91:873–81.

[178] Page DL, Caulfeld JB, Kastor JA, et al. Myocardial changes associated with cardiogenic shock. N Engl J Med 1971;285:133–7.

[179] Gacioch GM, Ellis SG, Lee L, et al. Cardiogenic shock complicating acute myocardial infarction: the use of coronary angioplasty and the integration of the new support devices into patient management. J Am Coll Cardiol 1992;19(3):647–53.

[180] Goldberg RJ, Samad NA, Yarzebski J, et al. Temporal trends in cardiogenic shock complicating acute myocardial infarction. N Engl J Med 1999;340:1162–8.

[181] Holmes DR, Berger PB, Hochman JS. Cardiogenic shock in patients with acute ischemic syndromes with and without ST-segment elevation. Circulation 1999;100:2067–73.

[182] Hasdai D, Califf RM, Thompson TD, et al. Predictors of cardiogenic shock after thrombolytic therapy for acute myocardial infarction. J Am Coll Cardiol 2000;35:136–43.

[183] Bowers TR, O'Neill WW, Grines C, et al. Effect of reperfusion on biventricular function and survival after right ventricular infarction. N Engl J Med 1998;338:933–40.

[184] Hochman JS, Buller CE, Sleeper LA, et al. Cardiogenic shock complicating acute myocardial infarction—etiologies, management and outcome: a report from the SHOCK trial registry. Should we emergently revascularize occluded coronaries for cardiogenic shock? J Am Coll Cardiol 2000;36(3 Suppl A):1063–70.

[185] Antoniucci D, Valenti R, Santoro GM, et al. Systematic direct angioplasty and stent supported direct angioplasty therapy for cardiogenic shock complicating acute myocardial infarction: in-hospital and long-term survival. J Am Coll Cardiol 1998;31:294–300.

[186] Bates ER, Topol EJ. Limitations of thrombolytic therapy for acute myocardial infarction complicated by congestive heart failure and cardiogenic shock. J Am Coll Cardiol 1991;18:1077–84.

[187] Samuels LE, Eduardo SD. Management of acute cardiogenic shock. Cardiol Clin 2003;21:43–9.

[188] Scheidt S, Wilner G, Mueller H, et al. Intra-aortic balloon counterpulsation in cardiogenic shock. N Engl J Med 1973;288:979–84.

[189] Waksman R, Weiss AT, Gotsman MS, et al. Intraaortic balloon counterpulsation improves survival in cardiogenic shock complicating acute myocardial infarction. Eur Heart J 1993;14:71–4.

[190] Gruppo Italiano per lo Studio della Streptokinasi. GISSI-2: a factorial randomized trial of alteplase versus streptokinase and heparin versus no heparin among 12,490 patients with acute myocardial infarction. Lancet 1990;336:65–71.

[191] Goldman L. Cost and quality of life: thrombolysis and primary angioplasty. J Am Coll Cardiol 1995;25(Suppl):38S–41S.

[192] Berger PB, Ellis SG, Holmes DR, et al. Relationship between delay in performing direct coronary angioplasty and early clinical outcome in patients with acute myocardial infarction: Results from the global use of strategies to open occluded arteries in Acute Coronary Syndromes (GUSTO-IIb) trial. Circulation 1999;100:14–20.

[193] Gacioch GM, Ellis SG, Lee L, et al. Cardiogenic shock complicating acute myocardial infarction: the use of coronary angioplasty and the integration of the new support devices into patient management. J Am Coll Cardiol 1992;19:647–53.

[194] Hochman JS, Sleeper LA, White HD, et al. One year survival following early revascularization for cardiogenic shock. JAMA 2001;285(2):190–2.

[195] DeWood MA, Notske RN, Hensley GR, et al. Intraaortic balloon counterpulsation with and without reperfusion for myocardial infarction shock. Circulation 1980;61(6):1105–12.

[196] Berger PB, Holmes DR, Stebbins AL, et al. Impact of an aggressive invasive catheterization and revascularization strategy on mortality in patients with cardiogenic shock in the Global Utilization of Streptokinase and Tissue Plasminogen Activator for Occluded Coronary Arteries (GUSTO-I) trial: an observational study. Circulation 1997;96:122–7.

[197] Hochman JS, Menon V, Connery C, et al. Outcome of patients undergoing cardiac surgery during hospitalization for cardiogenic shock complicating acute myocardial infarction. Circulation 1997;96:2431A.

[198] Mancini DM, Beniaminovitz A, Levin H, et al. Low incidence of myocardial recovery after left ventricular assist device implantation in patients with chronic heart failure. Circulation 1998; 98(22):2383–9.

[199] Dang NC, Topkara VK, Leacche M, et al. Left ventricular assist device implantation after acute anterior wall myocardial infarction and cardiogenic shock: a two-center study. J Thorac Cardiovasc Surg 2005;130(3):693–8.

[200] Lowe JE, Anstadt MP, Van Tright P, et al. First successful bridge to cardiac transplantation using direct mechanical ventricular actuation. Ann Thorac Surg 1991;52(6):1237–43.

[201] Loisance D, Deleuze M, Hillion ML, et al. The real impact of mechanical bridge strategy in patients with severe acute infarction. ASAIO Trans 1990; 36:M135–7.

[202] Levin HR, Burkhoff D, Oz MC, et al. Reversal of chronic ventricular dilation in patients with end-stage cardiomyopathy by prolonged mechanical unloading. Circulation 1995; 91:2717–20.

[203] Nakatani T, Takano H, Noda H, et al. Therapeutic effect of a left ventricular assist device on acute myocardial infarction evaluated by magnetic resonance imaging. Trans Am Soc Artif Intern Organs 1986;32:201–6.

[204] Oz MC, Rose EA, Slater J, et al. Malignant ventricular arrhythmias are well tolerated in patients receiving long-term left ventricular assist devices. J Am Coll Cardiol 1994;24:1688–91.

[205] Maggioni AP, Zuanetti G, Franzosi MG, et al. Prevalence and prognostic significance of ventricular arrhythmias after acute myocardial infarction in the fibrinolytic era, GISSI-2 results. Circulation 1993;87:312–22.

[206] Ratcliffe MB, Bavaria JE, Wenger RK, et al. Left ventricular mechanics of ejecting postischemic hearts during left ventricular circulatory assistance. J Thorac Cardiovasc Surg 1991;101(2): 245–55.

[207] DeRose JJ, Argenziano M, Sun BC, et al. Implantable left ventricular assist devices: an evolving long-term cardiac replacement therapy. Ann Surg 1997; 226:461–8.

[208] Oz MC, Goldstein DJ, Pepino P, et al. Screening scale predicts patients successfully receiving long-term, implantable left ventricular assist devices. Circulation 1995;92(Suppl II):169–73.

[209] Argenziano M, Choudhri AF, Moazami N, et al. A randomized, placebo controlled trial of inhaled nitric oxide in LVAD recipients with pulmonary hypertension. Ann Thorac Surg 1998;65:340–5.

[210] DiDonato M, Sabatier M, Dor V, et al. Effects of the Dor procedure on left ventricular dimension and shape and geometric correlates of mitral regurgitation one year after surgery. J Thorac Cardiovasc Surg 2001;121:91–6.

[211] Ingels NB. Myocardial fiber architecture and left ventricular function. Technol Health Care 1997;5: 45–52.

[212] Yamaguchi A, Adachi H, Kawahito K, et al. Left ventricular reconstruction benefits patients with dilated ischemic cardiomyopathy. Ann Thorac Surg 2005;79:456–61.

[213] Athanasuleas CL, Buckberg GD, Stanley AW, et al. Surgical ventricular restoration in the treatment of congestive heart failure due to post-infarction ventricular dilation. J Am Coll Cardiol 2004; 44(7):1439–45.

[214] Cooley DA, Frazier OH, Duncan JM, et al. Intracavitary repair of ventricular aneurysm and regional dyskinesia. Ann Surg 1992;215:417–23.

[215] DiDonato M, Sabatier M, Dor V, et al. Akinetic versus dyskinetic postinfarction scar: relation to surgical outcome in patients undergoing endoventricular circular patch plasty repair. J Am Coll Cardiol 1997;29:1569–75.

[216] DiDonato M, Sabatier M, Toso A, et al. Regional myocardial performance of non-ischemic zones remote from anterior wall left ventricular aneurysm: effects of aneursmectomy. Eur Heart J 1995;16: 1285–92.

ELSEVIER
SAUNDERS

Heart Failure Clin 3 (2007) 211–228

HEART
FAILURE
CLINICS

Revascularization in Heart Failure: Coronary Bypass or Percutaneous Coronary Intervention?

Sorin V. Pusca, MD, John D. Puskas, MD*

Emory University School of Medicine, Atlanta, GA, USA

Coronary artery disease (CAD) is currently the single most common cause of heart failure in adults [1]. The prognosis of patients who have severe CAD and left ventricular (LV) dysfunction remains poor despite new medical management algorithms [2–6]. Patients who have heart failure symptoms and a large area of ischemic myocardium treated medically may have a 5-year mortality as high as 60% [7]. Such patients often show marked improvement in symptoms and ventricular function following revascularization.

Baseline left ventricular ejection fraction (LVEF) is the single most powerful variable predictive of mortality after revascularization for acute myocardial infarction [8]. Its usefulness in selecting patients who have chronic disease for revascularization may not be as great, however. As an indicator of depressed LV function, ejection fraction alone does not distinguish between myocardium that is depressed because of reversible ischemia (ie, hibernating myocardium) and that which is replaced by fibrosis and scarring after previous myocardial infarction. There is increasing evidence that chronic LV dysfunction resulting from hibernating myocardium in patients who have severe multivessel disease is not uncommon [9]. Furthermore, even if some studies suggest that revascularization, particularly early revascularization (less than 6 months after testing), could help all patients who have decreased LVEF and

coronary artery disease regardless of myocardial viability [10], observational evidence suggests that myocardial revascularization results in stabilization or even improvement in ventricular function most commonly in patients who have viable, hibernating myocardium [11,12].

This article focuses primarily on the use of coronary artery bypass grafting (CABG) in CAD patients who have low LVEF (with or without congestive symptoms) and compares it with percutaneous coronary interventions (PCI) in this setting. Alternative modalities for the surgical treatment of ischemic heart failure, such as heart transplantation, surgical ventricular restoration, the Dor procedure, cardiomyoplasty, and the use of mechanical assist device for destination therapy, are not addressed in this article.

Results of coronary artery bypass grafting in patients who have low left ventricular ejection fraction

Many retrospective studies [13–17] and a large meta-analysis [18] have investigated the use of CABG in patients who have low LVEF. Several more recent studies are summarized in Table 1 [19–25]. Most of these document an operative mortality between 5% and 12% and a 5-year survival ranging from 60% to 80%.

One of the largest retrospective studies of CABG in patients who had advanced left ventricular dysfunction came from Emory University [26]. The study investigated short- and long-term survival and relief of angina among all patients who underwent cardiac catheterization followed by primary CABG at Emory University Hospitals from January 1981 to December 1995. A total of 11,830 patients were identified and stratified in

* Corresponding author. Emory Heart Center, Division of Cardiothoracic Surgery, Emory University School of Medicine, Emory Crawford Long Hospital, 6th Floor Medical Office Tower, 550 Peachtree Street NE, Atlanta, GA 30308.

E-mail address: john.puskas@emoryhealthcare.org (J.D. Puskas).

Table 1
Hospital mortality and long-term survival in patients who had low left ventricular ejection fraction treated by coronary artery bypass grafting in several recent series

Study	N	Age (mean or median, y)	EF (mean or median, y)	Hospital mortality	Follow-up duration	Follow-up survival
Shapira et al 1995 [21]	74	68.2	≤30%	NA	Cohort survival at 1, 2, 3, 4, 5, 6, 7 y	96%, 93.2%, 91.9%, 87.8%, 86.5%, 83.8%, 83.8%, 71%
Elefteriades et al 1997 [31]	135	66.5	23.6%	5.2%	Cohort survival at 1, 3, 4.5 y	87%, 81%, 71%
Trachiotis et al 1998 [26]	Group 1 = 156 patients, Group 2 = 588 patients	60	Group 1, EF <25%; Group 2, EF 25%–34%	Group 1, 3.8%; Group 2, 3.4%	Cohort survival at 1, 5, 7 y	Group 1: 90%, 64%, 49%; Group 2: 91.1%, 79.5%, 58.4%
Tjan et al 2000 [40]	51	63	16%	11.8%	45 months (1-y follow-up result)	71.9%
Veenhuyzen et al 2001 [27]	1870	61	28%	NA	1.8 y	81.6% (not including hospital mortality)
Lorusso et al 2001 [20]	120	60	28%	1.6%	Cohort survival at 5, 8 y	80%, 60%
Bouchart et al 2001 [25]	141	63.3	<22.2%	7%	Cohort survival at 2, 5, 7 y	84%, 70%, 50%
O'Connor et al 2002 [29]	343	63	29%	NA	5 y	61%
Carr et al 2002 [24]	86	65	18%	11%	Cohort survival at 5, 10 y	65%, 33%
Nishi et al 2003 [32]	42	66	23.8%	2.4%	32 mo	83%
Sawada et al 2003 [42]	95	60	33%	2.1%	4.9 y	62%
Ascione et al 2003 [22]	250	65	<30%	4%	Cohort survival at 1, 3 y	90%, 84%
Goldstein et al 2003 [23]	100	67	26%	3%	1 y	85%
Appoo et al 2004 [19]	430	64.5	<30%	4.6%	5 y	77.7%
DeRose et al 2005 [38]	544	65.2	≤25	5.5%	Cohort survival at 1, 5, 10 y	85%, 68%, 45%
Darwazah et al 2006 [30]	150	56.1 (OPCAB); 58.7 (ONCAB)	27.5% (OPCAB); 30.1% (ONCAB)	6.1% (OPCAB); 10.7% (ONCAB)	NA	NA
Hillis et al 2006 [50]	379	69	<35%	5.5%	3 y	81%

Abbreviations: NA, not applicable; ONCAB, on pump coronary artery bypass; OPCAB, off pump coronary artery bypass.

four groups: group 1, LVEF less than 25% (156 patients); group 2, LVEF 25% to 34% (588 patients); group 3, LVEF 35% to 49% (2438 patients); and group 4, LVEF greater than or equal to 50% (8649 patients). The outcome data, collected prospectively and entered into a dedicated, computerized database, are presented in Table 2. The long-term follow-up was complete in 99% of patients. Several important conclusions could be drawn from that study: (1) Patients who have low LVEF can be candidates for surgical revascularization with low mortality (although double that of patients who have normal LVEF) and low complication rates. (2) Patients who had low LVEF tended to have low incidence of perioperative Q-wave myocardial infarction (MI), possibly an indication of how successful the liberal use of intra-aortic balloon pump (IABP) is in decreasing perioperative ischemia. (3) Patients who have low LVEF have an acceptable 5- and 7-year survival. (4) Survival beyond 7 years is poor (23% at 10 years for LVEF <25%) and likely dictated by the progress of heart failure (Fig. 1).

CABG in patients who have low LVEF can have a significant protective effect for sudden death [27]. The reduction in mortality from sudden death among 1870 patients who had CABG in the SOLVD trials compared with 3540 patients who did not have CABG ranged from 39% if a broad definition of sudden death was used (ie, death occurring within 4 hours of onset of symptoms and classified as arrhythmic irrespective of preceding signs and symptoms of heart failure)

to 46% if a narrow definition of sudden death was used (ie, death occurring within 4 hours of onset of symptoms and classified as arrhythmic without preceding signs and symptoms of heart failure). This benefit in reducing sudden death was most pronounced in patients who had the lowest LVEF (Table 3). This difference was not explained by differences in other major prognostic factors (ie, age, gender, LVEF, and New York Heart Association [NYHA] functional class). Yusuf and Zucker [28] performed a meta-analysis of seven randomized controlled trials (RCTs) completed before 1994 that compared a strategy of initial CABG to a strategy of initial medical treatment of CAD. In a subset of 522 patients who had LVEF less than 50%, CABG offered a 10.6-month survival advantage at 5 years (statistically significant extension of life; $P < .001$). Only one third of these patients had LVEF less than 40%; the survival benefit was larger in patients who had lower LVEF, and 23% of patients assigned to initial medical treatment underwent CABG at 5-year follow-up.

O'Connor and colleagues [29] compared long-term outcomes in patients who had ischemic cardiomyopathy and low LVEF in 339 patients who underwent CABG versus 1052 patients who were treated medically from 1969 to 1994. The 5-year survival was 60% with CABG and 40% with medical treatment. Unadjusted, event-free, and risk-adjusted survival strongly favored CABG over medical therapy after 30 days to more than 10 years ($P < .001$). Furthermore, the

Table 2
Comparison of early and late outcomes for patients who have decreased versus normal ejection fraction

Variable	Group 1 (N = 156)	Group 2 (N = 588)	Group 3 (N = 2438)	Group 4 (N = 8649)	P
Average LVEF	0.19 ± 0.04	0.29 ± 0.03	0.42 ± 0.04	0.63 ± 0.09	<.0001
IABP use	10.7% (13)	10.6% (46)	6.5% (94)	3.7% (156)	<.0001
Hospital outcomes					
Mortality (N)	3.8% (6)	3.4% (20)	3.0% (72)	1.6% (134)	<.0001
Q-wave MI (N)	0% (0)	2% (12)	2% (48)	2.7% (231)	.04
Stroke (N)	2.6% (4)	2.9% (17)	2.2% (54)	1.4% (124)	.004
Length of stay (d)	9.2 ± 5.8	10.5 ± 10.9	9.1 ± 7.8	8.4 ± 6.4	<.0001
Late outcomes					
Time to follow-up (y)	5.8 ± 3.7	6.5 ± 4.2	7.2 ± 4.4	8.1 ± 4.8	<.0001
5-y survival (N)	64.4% (72)	71% (289)	82% (379)	89.6% (781)	<.0001
7-y survival (N)	49.1% (42)	58.4% (186)	73.3% (1012)	84.2% (4351)	<.0001
Angina during follow-up (N)	40% (31)	37% (122)	31% (532)	33% (2263)	.05

Abbreviations: IABP, intra-aortic balloon pump; MI, myocardial infarction.
Data from Trachiotis GD, Weintraub WS, Johnston TS, et al. Coronary artery bypass grafting in patients with advanced left ventricular dysfunction. Ann Thorac Surg 1998;66:1632–9.

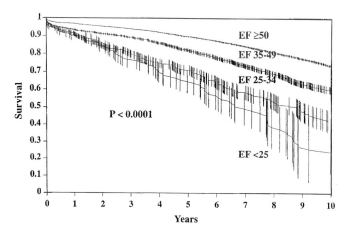

Fig. 1. Survival after CABG in patients who have sequentially decreased LVEF. (*From* Trachiotis GD, Weintraub WS, Johnston TS, et al. Coronary artery bypass grafting in patients with advanced left ventricular dysfunction. Ann Thorac Surg 1998;66:1635.)

survival curves diverge significantly for 5 to 10 years, suggesting an increased protective effect of CABG with time (Figs. 2–4).

The use of off-pump techniques may result in better survival [27], particularly if the patients have symptomatic heart failure, diabetes, or chronic obstructive pulmonary disease (COPD). Moreover, off pump coronary artery bypass (OPCAB) is associated with lower overall morbidity (19.7% versus 35.7%, $P = .01$), albeit with a lower number of grafts (2.0 ± 0.9 versus 3.4 ± 0.7, $P < .001$) in some studies [30].

Several authors [31,32] have shown that CABG in the setting of hibernating myocardium and low ejection fraction can result in rapid improvement of ejection fraction and symptoms (Table 4, Figs. 5–7).

Patient selection for coronary artery bypass grafting in the setting of low left ventricular ejection fraction

A key factor in obtaining good results with CABG in the setting of low LVEF is patient selection. The risk for CABG in the setting of LV dysfunction has historically been high. In 1983, Hochberg and colleagues [33] studied 466 patients who had LVEF less than 40% and found that overall perioperative mortality increased from 11% in patients who had LVEF between 20% and 39%, to 37% in patients who had LVEF less than 20%. Results of CABG improved dramatically over the last 2 decades, with significantly lower incidence of perioperative MI and early death. These improved outcomes are attributed to advances in myocardial protection (use of

Table 3

Reduction of sudden death risk with coronary artery bypass grafting by degree of left ventricular dysfunction in 1870 patients enrolled in the Studies of Left Ventricular Dysfunction trials

Baseline LVEF (No. of patients)	Limited definition (95% confidence limits)		Broad definition (95% confidence limits)	
	Absolute reduction[a]	Relative reduction (%)	Absolute reduction[a]	Relative reduction (%)
>0.30 (n = 1994)	−1.0* (−1.6 to −0.4)	−52* (−72 to −19)	−1.0* (−1.7 to −0.4)	−40* (−59 to −13)
0.25 to 0.30 (n = 1883)	−1.1* (−1.8 to −0.3)	−44* (−64 to −13)	−1.4* (−2.5 to −0.4)	−39* (−58 to −11)
<0.25 (n = 1532)	−1.6* (−2.8 to −0.5)	−38* (−58 to −9)	−1.7* (−3.2 to −0.3)	−33* (−53 to −6)

[a] Rate per 100 person-years.
* $P < .01$.

Data from Veenhuyzen GD, Singh SN, McAreavey D, et al. Prior coronary artery bypass surgery and risk of death among patients with ischemic left ventricular dysfunction. Circulation. 2001;104:1489–93.

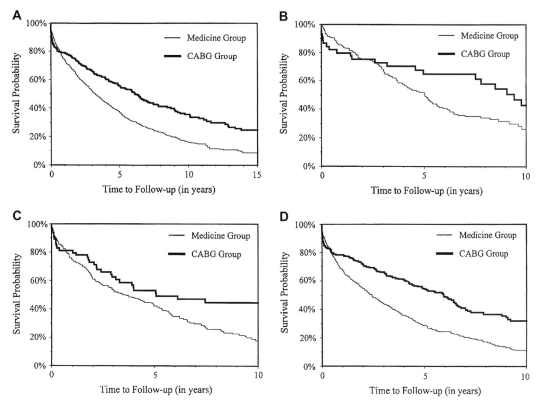

Fig. 2. (*A–D*) Unadjusted survival for patients who had low LVEF in Duke Cardiovascular Disease Databank. (*From* O'Connor CM, Velazquez EJ, Gardner LH, et al. Comparison of coronary artery bypass grafting versus medical therapy on long-term outcome in patients with ischemic cardiomyopathy. [A 25-year experience from the Duke Cardiovascular Disease Databank]. Am J Cardiol 2002;90:105; with permission.)

blood cardioplegia, retrograde continuous cardioplegia for myocardial preservation and resuscitation), surgical technique (the advent of off-pump CABG) and perioperative management (elective operation, stabilization using pre-, intra-, and postoperative IABP).

Ten years after Hochberg and colleagues [33], Hausmann and colleagues [34] investigated 224 patients who had LVEF between 10% and 30% and found an overall operative mortality of 8.9%. Univariate analysis found that within this group of patients who had depressed ventricular function the LVEF was not related to mortality. Similarly, Kaul and colleagues [35], analyzing 210 patients who had LVEF of 20% or less, found an operative mortality of 10%.

An excellent analysis of risk factors for perioperative mortality after CABG in patients who had low LVEF was performed by Argenziano and colleagues in 1999 [36]. The authors used the CABG Patch trial [37] that included 900 patients

younger then 80 years of age, with LVEF less than 36%, and an abnormal signal-averaged ECG (that would place them at a higher risk for arrhythmia after surgery), randomized to either CABG alone or CABG plus an automated implantable cardioverter defibrillator insertion. Perioperative mortality was defined broadly as death within 30 days of CABG or death within 90 days of CABG if continually hospitalized. Overall mortality was 5.6% Perioperative mortality rates by heart failure classification and angina symptoms are presented in Table 5. Two variables were significantly associated with perioperative mortality: NYHA class III/IV increased risk 2.4 times (*P* = .018) and redo CABG increased risk 3.8 times (*P* = .001).

DeRose and colleagues [38] analyzed 544 consecutive patients who had LVEF of 25% or less who underwent CABG, developing a score based on preoperative factors that is predictive of long-term mortality in patients who have low LVEF

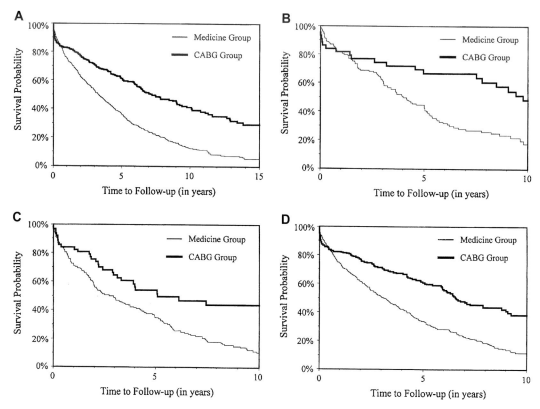

Fig. 3. (*A–D*) Adjusted survival for patients who had low LVEF in the Duke Cardiovascular Disease Databank. (*From* O'Connor CM, Velazquez EJ, Gardner LH, et al. Comparison of coronary artery bypass grafting versus medical therapy on long-term outcome in patients with ischemic cardiomyopathy. [A 25-year experience from the Duke Cardiovascular Disease Databank]. Am J Cardiol 2002;90:106; with permission.)

undergoing CABG. The score was named HAVOC for the risk factors involved (past congestive heart failure [CHF], age, peripheral Vascular disease, emergency operation, and COPD). The HAVOC score is defined:

$$HAVOC = 0.430 \text{ (if past CHF)}$$
$$+ 0.049 \text{ (age in years)}$$
$$+ 0.507 \text{ (if peripheral vascular disease)}$$
$$+ 0.580 \text{ (if emergency operation)}$$
$$+ 0.366 \text{ (if COPD)}$$

The 3-day mortality and 5-year survival rates for quartile classes are summarized in Table 6 and in Fig. 8.

An excellent study of CABG outcomes in patients who had low LVEF was performed by Topkara and colleagues [39]. The authors analyzed 55,515 patients who had CABG entered in the New York State Cardiac Surgery database between 1997 and 1999; 2442 patients had an LVEF less than 20%. The in-hospital mortality for this late class that had significantly more comorbidities at operation was a remarkable 6.5%. Eight clinical risk factors for adverse outcomes were identified: age, female gender, renal failure on dialysis, hepatic failure, CHF symptoms on admission, emergent operation, previous myocardial infarction within 6 hours, and reoperation (Table 7).

Other risk factors reported to be predictive of increased mortality after CABG in the setting of low LVEF are high left ventricular end diastolic pressure, elevated pulmonary artery pressures, and center experience [40].

Myocardial viability studies [41] can help identify classes of patients who have high risk for surgery and who derive little benefit from revascularization. Sawada and colleagues [42] investigated 95 patients who had CABG in the setting of low LV dysfunction and who had preoperative dobutamine

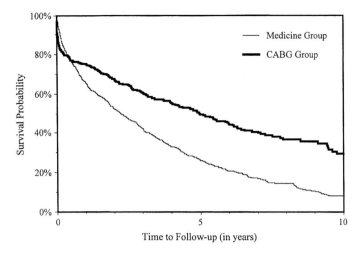

Fig. 4. Event-free survival for patients who had low LVEF in the Duke Cardiovascular Disease Databank. (*From* O'Connor CM, Velazquez EJ, Gardner LH, et al. Comparison of coronary artery bypass grafting versus medical therapy on long-term outcome in patients with ischemic cardiomyopathy. [A 25-year experience from the Duke Cardiovascular Disease Databank]. Am J Cardiol 2002;90:106; with permission.)

stress echocardiography to assess myocardial viability. Patients who had little myocardial viability (low-dose dobutamine score ≥2.5) had a 3-year survival of only 37%, whereas patients who had extensive myocardial viability (score <2) had a 5-year survival of 76% (Fig. 9). Some authors [43] have obtained excellent results guided only by clinical judgment, however, without the use of myocardial viability studies.

Direct comparison of coronary artery bypass grafting and percutaneous coronary intervention

A large number of RCTs have compared CABG and PCI outcomes for the treatment of CAD in general. Although some early data seemed to suggest equivalence for the two approaches, long-term follow-up and meta-analyses of multiple trials show that CABG offers a long-term survival advantage, particularly in patients who have multivessel disease [44,45].

Patients who had low LVEF were traditionally considered poor candidates for PCI. The advent of stents and perfusion catheters decreased significantly the incidence of acute vessel closure and infarction. PCI can be performed today in patients who have low LVEF with acceptable mortality (even if higher than in patients who have normal LVEF): in-hospital and 1-year mortality of 3.0% and 11% for LVEF 40% or less versus 0.1% and 1.9% for LVEF 50% or greater [46]. Furthermore, PCI for a patient who has low LVEF is not generally an ambulatory procedure but has an average hospital stay of 4.3 to 7 days [47,48].

In contrast with other subsets of patients who have CAD, comparison of PCI and CABG for revascularization of patients who have left ventricular dysfunction remains difficult because of

Table 4
Improvement in left ventricular ejection fraction and New York Heart Association class after coronary artery bypass grafting in patients who had left ventricular dysfunction

Study	N	Age (y)	Follow-up duration	LVEF preoperative	LVEF postoperative	NYHA preoperative	NYHA postoperative
Nishi et al 2003 [32]	42	66 ± 9.3	32 ± 26 mo	23.8% ± 4.5%	35.3% ± 8.5% (P<.05)	2.6 ± 0.7	1.1 ± 0.3
Elefteriades et al 1997 [31]	135	66.5 (42–87)	29 mo (1–89)	24%	34%	2.9	1.5 (P<.01)

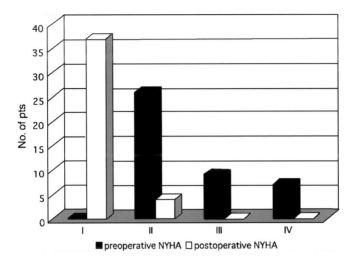

Fig. 5. Preoperative and postoperative symptom status for congestive heart failure (NYHA classification) in operative survivors showing number of patients in each group. (*From* Nishi H, Miyamoto S, Takanashi S, et al. Complete revascularization in patients with severe left ventricular dysfunction. Ann Thorac Cardiovasc Surg 2003;9:115. Copyright © 2003 by the Editorial Board of the Annals of Thoracic and Cardiovasculor Surgery. All rights reserved.)

lack of extensive data. Several limited series and only one RCT have addressed this question.

O'Keefe and colleagues [48] compared outcomes for 100 consecutive patients treated with CABG with those of a cohort of 100 patients (matched for age, sex, and LVEF) treated with multivessel angioplasty, all with LVEF less than or equal to 40% (mean LVEF 31%), from February 1985 to September 1988. Hospital mortality was similar (5% CABG versus 3% angioplasty). There was a trend in long-term outcome for better survival with CABG, 76% versus 67% at 5 years ($P<.09$) (Fig. 10). This absolute difference of almost 10% was not statistically significant because of the small number of patients (18 patients for CABG and 17 patients for PCI). Cardiac event-free survival, however, was statistically superior in CABG patients: 76% versus 46% ($P<.01$) (Fig. 11). Symptomatic improvement was also superior in CABG patients with most patients (88%) being in NYHA class I status after CABG but only two thirds (68%) after PCI; 11 patients were in NYHA class III/IV after PCI versus only 1 patient after CABG (Table 8). The

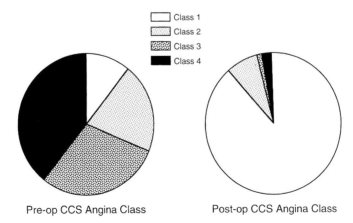

Fig. 6. Change in angina status following CABG in 135 patients who had LVEF less than or equal to 30%. CCS, Canadian Cardiovascular Society. (*From* Elefteriades JA, Morales DLS, Gradel C, et al. Results of coronary artery bypass grafting by a single surgeon in patients with left ventricular ejection fractions ≤ 30%. Am J Cardiol 1997;79:1576; with permission.)

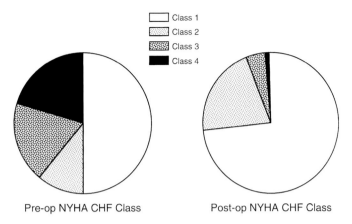

Pre-op NYHA CHF Class   Post-op NYHA CHF Class

Fig. 7. Change in CHF status following CABG in 135 patients who had LVEF less than or equal to 30%. (*From* Elefteriades JA, Morales DLS, Gradel C, et al. Results of coronary artery bypass grafting by a single surgeon in patients with left ventricular ejection fractions ≤ 30%. Am J Cardiol 1997;79:1576; with permission.)

superior results of CABG were attributed to the more complete revascularization achieved with CABG: 18% of patients treated with CABG had incomplete revascularization versus 63% of those treated with PCI, $P < .001$.

Berger and colleagues [49] investigated a subset of 176 patients from the largest RCT of CABG versus PCI, the BARI trial (Bypass Angioplasty Revascularization Trial, completed between 1988 and 1991). Among this subset of patients who had multivessel disease and LVEF less than 50%, the 7-year survival was 70% after percutaneous transluminal coronary angioplasty (PTCA) and 74% after CABG ($P = .6$) [50]. The average LVEF of patients who had LVEF less than 50% was 41% and the symptomatic status of these patients was not described.

Toda and colleagues [47] investigated 117 consecutive patients who had severe LV dysfunction ($15\% \leq LVEF \leq 30\%$, mean LVEF 24%)

who underwent either CABG (N = 69) or PCI (N = 48) between 1992 and 1997. Mortality was similar at 30 days and 3 years (7% CABG versus 8% PCI and 27% versus 33%, $P = .39$), but the PCI group follow-up was significantly shorter then the CABG group (38 ± 14 months versus 51 ± 19 months). Moreover, there was a significantly better 3-year cardiac event-free survival after CABG (52% versus 25%, $P = .0011$), largely attributable to improved survival in patients who had proximal left anterior descending artery (LAD) disease and younger patients treated with CABG. There was a marked and statistically significant improvement in LVEF with CABG (from 25% ± 4% to 37% ± 15%, $P < .0001$) but no improvement with PCI (26% ± 4% to 30% ± 13%, P not significant), and again, more complete target vessel revascularization (incomplete revascularization 16% with CABG and 52% with PCI, $P < .0001$). This study did not address

Table 5
Perioperative mortality rates by heart failure and angina symptoms

NYHA heart failure class	Mortality for CCS angina class			
	No angina	I/II	III/IV	Total
No heart failure	0.013 (80)	0.031 (163)	0.044 (182)	0.033 (425)
I/II	0.048 (63)	0.103 (78)	0.091 (66)	0.082 (207)
III/IV	0.074 (68)	0.089 (45)	0.074 (95)	0.077 (208)
Total	0.043 (211)	0.059 (286)	0.061 (343)	0.056 (840)

Values in parentheses indicate number of patients in each group. Data were missing for 60 patients. There were 47 perioperative deaths among the 840 remaining patients.

Abbreviation: CCS, Canadian Cardiovascular Society.

Data from Argenziano M, Spotnitz HM, Whang W, et al. Risk stratification for coronary bypass surgery in patients with left ventricular dysfunction analysis of the coronary artery bypass grafting patch trial database. Circulation 1999;100(Suppl II):II-119–24.

Table 6
Short- and long-term outcome based on HAVOC score
for patients who have left ventricular ejection fraction
less than or equal to 25%

HAVOC score	30-d mortality	5-y survival
HAVOC≤3.18	3.0%	82.3%
3.18<HAVOC<3.59	2.9%	78.2%
3.59<HAVOC<4.05	5.1%	65.5%
HAVOC>4.05	10.9%	45.5%
P value	P = .011	P<.0001

Data from DeRose Jr JJ, Toumpoulis IK, Balaram
SK, et al. Preoperative prediction of long-term survival
after coronary artery bypass grafting in patients with
low left ventricular ejection fraction. J Thorac
Cardiovasc Surg 2005;129:314–21.

any differences in NYHA class status. These midterm results did not evaluate whether significantly
better LVEF in CABG patients could translate to
superior long-term survival.

Brener and colleagues [51] performed a propen-
sity score analysis of 6033 patients who underwent
PCI or CABG at the Cleveland Clinic between
January 1995 and December 1999. There was

frequent use of GP IIb/IIIa inhibitors and stents
in the PCI group. A total of 627 patients had an
LVEF less than or equal to 30% (54 patients
had PCI and 573 had CABG, P<.0001). This
study represents one of the largest analyses in
the field. Five-year survival was 63% for PCI
and 72% for CABG (adjusted hazard ratio for
mortality with PCI versus CABG 1.6, 95% CI
0.9–2.7, P = .09). The large 9% absolute survival
advantage at 5-year follow-up with CABG
showed only a trend toward statistical significance
because of the asymmetric size of these two
patient groups.

The AWESOME (Angina With Extremely
Serious Operative Mortality Evaluation) trial
[52], was a national prospective randomized study
of the Department of Veterans Affairs (VA)
designed to compare the long-term survival of
patients who had medically refractory myocardial
ischemia and increased risk factors for coronary
revascularization who were assigned to either
CABG or PCI. The primary endpoint of the study
was survival and the secondary endpoints were
unstable angina and repeat hospitalization,

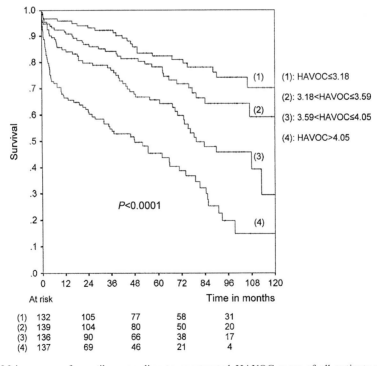

Fig. 8. Kaplan-Meier curves of quartiles according to constructed HAVOC score of all patients who had low EF
(<25%) undergoing CABG (n = 544). (*From* DeRose JJ Jr, Toumpoulis IK, Balaram SK, et al. Preoperative prediction
of long-term survival after coronary artery bypass grafting in patients with low left ventricular ejection fraction. J Thorac
Cardiovasc Surg 2005;129:318; with permission.)

Table 7
Independent predictors of in-hospital mortality in patients who have left ventricular ejection fraction less than 20%

Risk factor	Variable estimate	SE	P value	Odds ratio[a]	95% CI
Age	0.039	0.009	<.001	1.040	1.021–1.059
Female gender	0.546	0.185	.003	1.726	1.201–2.482
Renal failure on dialysis	1.417	0.426	.001	4.125	1.788–9.513
Hepatic failure	2.416	0.688	.001	11.203	2.907–43.175
CHF, this admission	0.488	0.196	.013	1.629	1.110–2.390
Emergent operation	1.165	0.341	.001	3.207	1.645–6.251
Previous MI <6 h	1.221	0.349	<.001	3.392	1.713–6.717
Reoperation	1.215	0.248	<.001	3.369	2.071–5.481

[a] OR for every 1-y increase in age. Hosmer-Lemeshow goodness-of-fit test: $P = .586$.

Data from Topkara VK, Cheema FH, Kesavaramanujam S, et al. Coronary artery bypass grafting in patients with low ejection fraction. Circulation. 2005;112(Suppl I):I-344–50.

catheterization, CABG, and/or PCI. It is the only RCT completed to date to include randomized CABG–PCI data comparison for patients who had low LVEF. The study enrolled at 16 VA centers across the United States from February 1995 to March 2000. It screened 22,662 patients and found 2431 clinically eligible patients; 781 were deemed appropriate candidates for randomization and 454 consented to randomization. The 327 patients who refused random allocation and elected either CABG or PCI were prospectively entered into a patient-choice registry. The 1650 patients

for whom physician consensus would not allow random allocation were entered prospectively into a physician-directed registry [53,54].

A total of 446 patients had LVEF less than 35%: 94 were randomized to CABG or PCI, 300 entered the physician-directed registry, and 52 entered the patient-choice registry. The outcomes for all the patients who had LVEF less than 35% were analyzed separately (Tables 9 and 10) [53]. The investigators concluded that "The results of the AWESOME study (including the only group of patients with EF < 35% randomly allocated

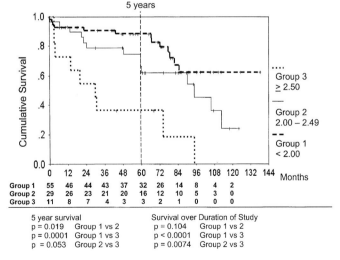

Fig. 9. Survival of three groups of patients who had extensive (group 1), intermediate (group 2), and limited (group 3) myocardial viability based on low-dose dobutamine stress echocardiogram wall motion scores. Two patients who had perioperative deaths are included. Log-rank *P* values comparing survival among the three groups at 5 years and for the complete duration of the study are shown at the bottom of the figure. (*From* Sawada S, Bapat A, Vaz D, et al. Incremental value of myocardial viability for prediction of long-term prognosis in surgically revascularized patients with left ventricular dysfunction. J Am Coll Cardiol 2003;42:2103; with permission.)

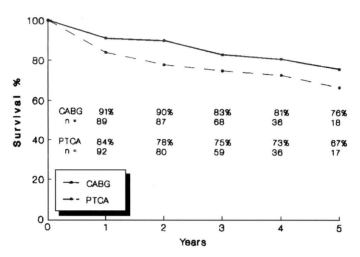

Fig. 10. Long-term survival (including in-hospital mortality) in CABG versus PTCA (*P* = .09). (*From* O'Keefe JH, Allan JJ, McCallister BD, et al. Angioplasty versus bypass surgery for multivessel coronary artery disease with left ventricular ejection fraction < 40%. Am J Cardiol 1993;71:898; with permission.)

to therapy with PCI versus CABG) suggest that the outcomes with PCI in the current era are similar to those with CABG for patients with acute coronary syndromes, even in the presence of low LVEFs." Unfortunately the results are presented only as percentages and one cannot calculate how many patients were included in each group; the number of patients in the randomized group is extremely small and the risk factors for the patients who were included in the small randomized group are not compared between groups. The largest proportion of patients who have low

LVEF is in the physician-directed registry. The results, similarly favorable in both groups, may be largely attributable to appropriate referral to CABG or PCI (eg, in the physician-directed registry in general 83% of patients who underwent CABG had CHF, whereas only 57% of patients who had PCI had CHF, *P*<.01). The use of arterial conduits that potentially could offer survival advantage was low overall in this study (left internal mammary artery [LIMA] 70%, right internal mammary artery 3.4%, and radial artery 2.8%). This figure represents a lower LIMA use then

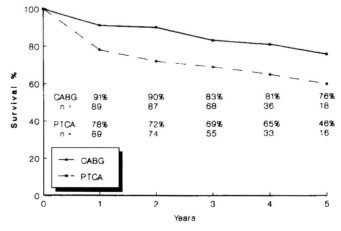

Fig. 11. Long-term event-free survival (freedom from death or infarction during follow-up) in CABG versus PTCA (*P*<.01). (*From* O'Keefe JH, Allan JJ, McCallister BD, et al. Angioplasty versus bypass surgery for multivessel coronary artery disease with left ventricular ejection fraction <40%. Am J Cardiol 1993;71:899; with permission.)

Table 8

Baseline and follow-up symptomatic status after coronary artery bypass grafting and percutaneous transluminal coronary angioplasty

Baseline and follow-up symptomatic status[a]

Class	Baseline procedure*		Follow-up (mean 3.5 years)**	
	CABG	PTCA	CABG	PTCA
I	12	21	88	68
II	6	16	11	21
III	20	17	1	8
IV	57	46	0	3

Two thirds of PTCA patients are in NYHA class II or above, whereas 90% of CABG patients are in NYHA class I.

Abbreviation: PTCA, percutaneous transluminal coronary angioplasty.

[a] New York Heart Association classification (except for class I defined as asymptomatic)

* $P < .001$ at baseline

** $P < .01$ at follow-up: CABG versus PTCA.

Data from O'Keefe JH, Allan JJ, McCallister BD, et al. Angioplasty versus bypass surgery for multivessel coronary artery disease with left ventricular ejection fraction <40%. Am J Cardiol 1993;71:897–901.

other recent studies [52] (EAST trial 86% and BARI trial 84% LIMA use). Furthermore, there was a 10% higher incidence of three-vessel disease in the CABG registry patients in this small series. The study did not include a meaningful number of women, which is a recognized limitation of VA trials, but which also could lead to artificially improved outcomes. Furthermore, the study included patients who had ongoing or very recent MI that could have potentially a larger amount of hibernating myocardium and less myocardial

scarring than patients who had low LVEF in a chronic setting.

It has been argued that generalization of conclusions from RCTs is inappropriate in many instances because the conclusions of such trials reliably apply only to the small percentage of patients enrolled in these trials. These patients are generally selected by virtue of being considered by common standards to be good candidates for both interventions tested. It is therefore not surprising to find limited differences in outcomes between randomly assigned groups of such patients. These results may not correctly inform clinicians about appropriate care for the large majority of patients seen in daily practice [44]. Furthermore, RCTs tend to include younger patients who have better cardiovascular risk profiles when compared with patients seen in practice, as the Euro Heart Survey showed [55].

Such an impression is confirmed by an analysis of the New York State databases [56] that included nearly 60,000 patients who underwent either CABG or PCI for CAD from January 1997 to December 2000 (9952 with LVEF less than 40% and either three-vessel disease or two-vessel disease involving the proximal LAD). This study was approximately concurrent with the AWESOME trial. Risk-adjusted hazard ratios for death in patients who had LVEF less than 40% after CABG compared with PCI were 0.64 in patients who had two-vessel disease and proximal LAD disease and in patients who had three-vessel disease and disease of nonproximal LAD, and 0.68 in patients who had three-vessel disease and disease of the proximal LAD. This finding represents a 30% to 40% relative increase in the risk for death for patients who had low LVEF treated with an initial strategy of multivessel PCI versus

Table 9

Coronary artery bypass grafting and percutaneous coronary intervention 36-month outcomes in the AWESOME trial and registry

	Randomized (%)		Physician directed (%)		Patient choice (%)	
	CABG	PCI	CABG	PCI	CABG	PCI
Survival	72	69	59	61	68	71
Survival free of unstable angina	41	37	42	41	42	43
Survival free of unstable angina or repeat revascularization	41	37	42	40	42	43

Data from Sedlis SP, Ramanathan KB, Morrison DA, and the Investigators of the Department of Veterans Affairs Cooperative Study #385, the Angina With Extremely Serious Operative Mortality Evaluation (AWESOME). Outcome of percutaneous coronary intervention versus coronary bypass grafting for patients with low left ventricular ejection fractions, unstable angina pectoris, and risk factors for adverse outcomes with bypass (the AWESOME randomized trial and registry). Am J Cardiol 2004;94:118–20.

Table 10
Hazard ratios for death after coronary artery bypass grafting as compared with percutaneous coronary intervention in patients who had left ventricular ejection fraction less than 40% and multivessel coronary artery disease in the New York State Databases 1997–2000

Extent of CAD	CABG (patients at risk)	PCI (patients at risk)	Hazard ratio (risk-adjusted)	95% CI
Two-vessel disease involving proximal LAD	1615	803	0.64	0.51–0.81
Three-vessel disease not involving proximal LAD	1196	342	0.64	0.48–0.87
Three-vessel disease involving proximal LAD	5597	399	0.68	0.54–0.85

Data from Hannan EL, Racz MJ, Walford G, et al. Long-term outcomes of coronary-artery bypass grafting versus stent implantation. N Engl J Med 2005;352:2174–83.

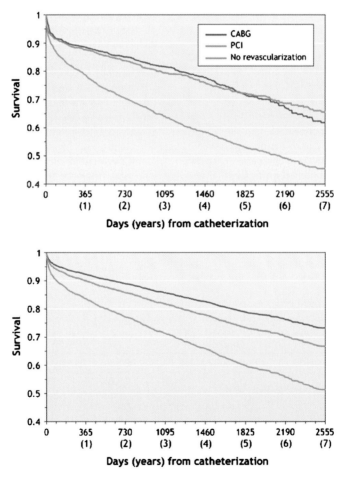

Fig. 12. Survival of patients who had heart failure, according to revascularization strategy. Upper panel shows crude survival; lower panel shows risk-adjusted survival. (*From* Tsuyuki RT, Shrive FM, Galbraith PD, et al. for the APPROACH Investigators. Revascularization in patients with heart failure. CMAJ, 2006;175(4):364; with permission.)

CABG (see Table 9). This real-world experience of a huge number of patients arguably provides a much more reliable and realistic guide for patient treatment than the super-selected small subset of patients randomized in the AWESOME trial.

An analysis of the Canadian APPROACH database (Alberta Provincial Project for Outcomes Assessment in Coronary Heart Disease) [57] that began in 1995 and followed patients for up to 7 years included 4228 patients who had heart failure who underwent a cardiac catheterization: 2538 patients underwent revascularization by CABG or PCI and 1690 patients were treated with medical management alone. No direct comparison between CABG and PCI was made. Risk-adjusted survival curves for CABG seem superior to PCI (adjusted hazard ratio for CABG 0.44, 95% CI 0.38–0.52 versus 0.58 for PCI, 95% CI 0.49–0.69, both calculated against medical management group) (Fig. 12).

Surgical revascularization for patients who have low LVEF remains a challenging procedure and in general should be attempted in centers able and willing to provide mechanical assist or heart transplant services. The oft-cited operative mortality of 5% to 8% is the mortality of centers with significant experience in handling such patients.

Summary

From the analysis of clinical series presented above we learn that selected patients who have low LVEF and CAD clearly benefit from coronary revascularization with CABG, and that CABG offers a 5-year survival of 60% to 70% and a life extension of close to a year at 5 years' follow-up compared with a strategy of initial medical management, with an average perioperative mortality between 5% to 8% in experienced hands (twice that of patients who have normal ejection fraction). Clinical improvement should be expected in most patients who undergo CABG. This is important for patients who have a limited life span that they could spend with a good functional status rather than being hospitalized for multiple repeat PCIs or symptomatic deterioration.

Clinical variables, the use of HAVOC score, and myocardial viability testing are tools that can help refine patient selection. The weight the clinical information available suggests that revascularization by CABG seems to be superior to PCI in most patients who have low ejection fraction, particularly in patients who have low LVEF and symptoms of angina. There are situations, however, in which PCI may be helpful, such as in patients who have low ejection fraction and one or more previous cardiac operations, or in those whose severe noncardiac comorbidities preclude major surgery.

References

[1] Bourassa MG, Gurne O, Bangdiwala SI, et al. Natural history and patterns of current practice in heart failure. The studies of left ventricular dysfunction (SOLVD) investigators. J Am Coll Cardiol 1993; 4(Suppl A):14A–9A.

[2] Anonymous (The CONSENSUS trial Study group). Effects of enalapril on mortality in severe congestive heart failure. N Engl J Med 1987;316: 1429–35.

[3] Anonymous (The SOLVD Investigators). Effect of enalapril on survival in patients with reduced left ventricular ejection fractions and congestive heart failure. N Engl J Med 1991;325:293–302.

[4] Packer M, Bristow MR, Cphn JN, et al. The effect of carvedilol on morbidity and mortality in patients with chronic heart failure. N Engl J Med 1996;334: 1349–55.

[5] Anonymous (MERIT-HF Study Group). Effect of metoprolol CR/XL in chronic heart failure: metoprolol CR/XL randomized intervention trial in congestive heart failure (MERIT-HF). Lancet 1999;353:2001–7.

[6] Pitt B, Zannad F, Remme WJ, et al. The effect of spironolactone on morbidity and mortality in patients with severe heart failure. Randomized aldactone evaluation study investigators. N Engl J Med 1999; 341:709–17.

[7] Miller WL, Tointon SK, Hodge DO, et al. Long-term outcome and the use of revascularization in patients with heart failure, suspected ischemic heart disease, and large reversible myocardial perfusion defects. Am Heart J 2002;143:904–9.

[8] Halkin A, Singh M, Nikolsky E, et al. Prediction of mortality after primary percutaneous coronary intervention for acute myocardial infarction the CADILLAC risk score. J Am Coll Cardiol 2005; 45:1397–405.

[9] Eagle KA, Guyton RA, The American College of Cardiology/American Heart Association Task Force on ACC/AHA PRACTICE GUIDELINES (Committee to Update the 1999 Guidelines for Coronary Artery Bypass Graft Surgery). ACC/AHA 2004 guideline update for coronary artery bypass graft surgery: a report of the American College of Cardiology/American Heart Association task force on practice guidelines developed in collaboration with the American association for thoracic surgery

and the society of thoracic surgeons. Circulation 2004;110:340–437.

[10] Tarakji KG, Brunken R, McCarthy PM, et al. Myocardial viability testing and the effect of early intervention in patients with advanced left ventricular systolic dysfunction. Circulation 2006;113: 230–7.

[11] Bourque JM, Hasselblad V, Velazquez EJ, et al. Revascularization in patients with coronary artery disease, left ventricular dysfunction, and viability: a meta-analysis. Am Heart J 2003;146:621–7.

[12] Allman KC, Shaw LJ, Hachamovitch R, et al. Myocardial viability testing and impact of revascularization on prognosis in patients with coronary artery disease and left ventricular dysfunction: a meta-analysis. J Am Coll Cardiol 2002;39:1151–8.

[13] Elefteriades JA, Tolis G, Levi E, et al. Coronary artery bypass grafting in severe left ventricular dysfunction: excellent survival with improved ejection fraction and functional state. J Am Coll Cardiol 1993;22:1411–7.

[14] Meluzín J, Cerný J, Frélich M, et al. Prognostic value of the amount of dysfunctional but viable myocardium in revascularized patients with coronary artery disease and left ventricular dysfunction. J Am Coll Cardiol 1998;32:912–20.

[15] Myers WO, Gersh BJ, Fisher LD, et al. Medical versus early surgical therapy in patients with triple-vessel disease and mild angina pectoris: a CASS registry study of survival. Ann Thorac Surg 1987;44: 471–86.

[16] Myers WO, Schaff HV, Gersh BJ, et al. Improved survival of surgically treated patients with triple vessel coronary artery disease and severe angina pectoris: a report from the Coronary Artery Surgery Study (CASS) registry. J Thorac Cardiovasc Surg 1989;97:487–95.

[17] Pagley PR, Beller GA, Watson DD, et al. Improved outcome after coronary bypass surgery in patients with ischemic cardiomyopathy and residual myocardial viability. Circulation 1997;96:793–800.

[18] Baker DW, Jones R, Hodges J, et al. Management of heart failure, III: the role of revascularization in the treatment of patients with moderate or severe left ventricular systolic dysfunction. JAMA 1994;272: 1528–34.

[19] Appoo J, Norris C, Merali S, et al. Long-term outcome of isolated coronary artery bypass surgery in patients with severe left ventricular dysfunction-Circulation 2004;110(Suppl II):II13–7.

[20] Lorusso R, LaCanna G, Ceconi C, et al. Long-term results of coronary artery bypass grafting procedure in the presence of left ventricular dysfunction and hibernating myocardium. Eur J Cardiothorac Surg 2001;20:937–48.

[21] Shapira I, Isakov A, Yakirevich V, et al. Long-term results of coronary artery bypass surgery in patients with severely depressed left ventricular function. Chest 1995;108:1546–50.

[22] Ascione R, Narayan P, Rogers CA, et al. Early and midterm clinical outcome in patients with severe left ventricular dysfunction undergoing coronary artery surgery. Ann Thorac Surg 2003;76(3): 793–9.

[23] Goldstein DJ, Beauford RB, Luk B, et al. Multivessel off-pump revascularization in patients with severe left ventricular dysfunction. Eur J Cardiothorac Surg 2003;24(1):72–80.

[24] Carr JA, Haithcock BE, Paone G, et al. Long-term outcome after coronary artery bypass grafting in patients with severe left ventricular dysfunction. Ann Thorac Surg 2002;74(5):1531–6.

[25] Bouchart F, Tabley A, Litzler PY, et al. Myocardial revascularization in patients with severe ischemic left ventricular dysfunction. Long term follow-up in 141 patients. Eur J Cardiothorac Surg 2001;20(6): 1157–62.

[26] Trachiotis GD, Weintraub WS, Johnston TS, et al. Coronary artery bypass grafting in patients with advanced left ventricular dysfunction. Ann Thorac Surg 1998;66:1632–9.

[27] Veenhuyzen GD, Singh SN, McAreavey D, et al. Prior coronary artery bypass surgery and risk of death among patients with ischemic left ventricular dysfunction. Circulation 2001;104:1489–93.

[28] Yusuf S, Zucker D. Effect of coronary artery bypass graft surgery on survival: overview of 10-year results from randomised trials by the Coronary Artery Bypass Graft Surgery Trialists Collaboration. Lancet 1994;344:563–70.

[29] O'Connor CM, Velazquez EJ, Gardner LH, et al. Comparison of coronary artery bypass grafting versus medical therapy on long-term outcome in patients with ischemic cardiomyopathy (a 25-year experience from the Duke Cardiovascular Disease Databank). Am J Cardiol 2002;90:101–7.

[30] Darwazah AK, Sham'a RAA, Hussein E, et al. Myocardial revascularization in patients with low ejection fraction ≤35%: effect of pump technique on early morbidity and mortality. J Card Surg 2006;21:22–7.

[31] Elefteriades JA, Morales DLS, Gradel C, et al. Results of coronary artery bypass grafting by a single surgeon in patients with left ventricular ejection fractions < 30%. Am J Cardiol 1997;79:1573–8.

[32] Nishi H, Miyamoto S, Takanashi S, et al. Complete revascularization in patients with severe left ventricular dysfunction. Ann Thorac Cardiovasc Surg 2003;9:111–6.

[33] Hochberg MS, Parsonnet V, Gielchinsky I, et al. Coronary artery bypass grafting in patients with drastic impairment of function of the left ventricle. J Thorac Cardiovasc Surg 1983;86:519–27.

[34] Hausmann H, Warnecke H, Ennker J, et al. Survival predictors in patients with a left ventricular ejection fraction of 10-30% receiving a coronary bypass: analysis of preoperative variables. Cardiovasc Surg 1993;2:558–62.

[35] Kaul EK, Agnihotri AK, Fields BL, et al. Coronary artery bypass grafting in patients with an ejection fraction of twenty percent or less. J Thorac Cardiovasc Surg 1996;111:1001–12.

[36] Argenziano M, Spotnitz HM, Whang W, et al. Risk stratification for coronary bypass surgery in patients with left ventricular dysfunction analysis of the coronary artery bypass grafting patch trial database. Circulation 1999;100(Suppl II):II119–24.

[37] Bigger JTfor the Coronary Artery Bypass Graft (CABG) Patch Trial Investigators. Prophylactic use of implanted cardiac defibrillators in patients at high risk for ventricular arrhythmias after coronary-artery bypass graft surgery. N Engl J Med 1997;337:1569–75.

[38] DeRose JJ Jr, Toumpoulis IK, Balaram SK, et al. Preoperative prediction of long-term survival after coronary artery bypass grafting in patients with low left ventricular ejection fraction. J Thorac Cardiovasc Surg 2005;129:314–21.

[39] Topkara VK, Cheema FH, Kesavaramanujam S, et al. Coronary artery bypass grafting in patients with low ejection fraction. Circulation 2005;112(Suppl I):I344–50.

[40] Tjan TDT, Kondruweit M, Scheld HH, et al. The bad ventricle—revascularization versus transplantation. J Thorac Cardiovasc Surg 2000;48:9–14.

[41] Afridi I, Grayburn PA, Panza JA, et al. Myocardial viability during dobutamine echocardiography predicts survival in patients with coronary artery disease and severe left ventricular systolic dysfunction. J Am Coll Cardiol 1998;32:921–6.

[42] Sawada S, Bapat A, Vaz D, et al. Incremental value of myocardial viability for prediction of long-term prognosis in surgically revascularized patients with left ventricular dysfunction. J Am Coll Cardiol 2003;42:2099–105.

[43] Mickleborough LL, Carson S, Tamariz M, et al. Results of revascularization in patients with severe left ventricular dysfunction. J Thorac Cardiovasc Surg 2000;119(3):550–7.

[44] Guyton RA. Coronary artery bypass is superior to drug-eluting stents in multivessel coronary artery disease. Ann Thorac Surg 2006;81:1949–57.

[45] Hoffman SN, TenBrook JA Jr, Wolf MP, et al. A meta-analysis of randomized controlled trials comparing coronary artery bypass graft with percutaneous transluminal coronary angioplasty: one- to eight-year outcomes. J Am Coll Cardiol 2003;41:1293–304.

[46] Keelan PC, Johnston JM, Koru-Sengul T, et al(for the Dynamic Registry Investigators). Comparison of in-hospital and one-year outcomes in patients with left ventricular ejection fractions <40%, 41% to 49%, and >50% having percutaneous coronary revascularization. Am J Cardiol 2003;91:1168–72.

[47] Toda K, Mackenzie K, Mehra MR, et al. Revascularization in severe ventricular dysfunction (15% < LVEF < 30%): a comparison of bypass grafting and percutaneous intervention. Ann Thorac Surg 2002;74:2082–7.

[48] O'Keefe JH, Allan JJ, McCallister BD, et al. Angioplasty versus bypass surgery for multivessel coronary artery disease with left ventricular ejection fraction <40%. Am J Cardiol 1993;71:897–901.

[49] Berger PB, Velianou JL, Vlachos HA, et alfor the BARI Investigators. Survival following coronary angioplasty versus coronary artery bypass surgery in anatomic subsets in which coronary artery bypass surgery improves survival compared with medical therapy results from the bypass angioplasty revascularization investigation (BARI). J Am Coll Cardiol 2001;38:1440–9.

[50] Hillis GS, Zehr KJ, Williams AW, et al. Outcome of patients with low ejection fraction undergoing coronary artery bypass grafting renal function and mortality after 3.8 years. Circulation 2006;114(Suppl I):I414–9.

[51] Brener SJ, Lytle BW, Casserly IP, et al. Propensity analysis of long-term survival after surgical or percutaneous revascularization in patients with multivessel coronary artery disease and high-risk features. Circulation 2004;109:2290–5.

[52] Morrison DA, Sethi G, Sacks J, et alFor the Investigators of the Department of Veterans Affairs Cooperative Study #385, the Angina With Extremely Serious Operative Mortality Evaluation (AWESOME). Percutaneous coronary intervention versus coronary artery bypass graft surgery for patients with medically refractory myocardial ischemia and risk factors for adverse outcomes with bypass: a multicenter, randomized trial. J Am Coll Cardiol 2001;38:143–9.

[53] Sedlis SP, Ramanathan KB, Morrison DA, et al. Outcome of percutaneous coronary intervention versus coronary bypass grafting for patients with low left ventricular ejection fractions, unstable angina pectoris, and risk factors for adverse outcomes with bypass (the awesome randomized trial and registry). Am J Cardiol 2004;94:118–20.

[54] Morrison DA, Sethi G, Sacks J, et alFor the Investigators of the Department of Veterans Affairs Cooperative Study #385, the Angina With Extremely Serious Operative Mortality Evaluation (AWESOME). . Percutaneous coronary intervention versus coronary bypass graft surgery for patients with medically refractory myocardial ischemia and risk factors for adverse outcomes with bypass the VA AWESOME multicenter registry: comparison with the randomized clinical trial. J Am Coll Cardiol 2002;39:266–73.

[55] Hordijk-Trion M, Lenzen M, Wijns W, et al. (for the EHS-CR Investigators). Patients enrolled in coronary intervention trials are not representative of

patients in clinical practice: results from the Euro Heart Survey on coronary revascularization. Eur Heart J 2006;27:671–8.

[56] Hannan EL, Racz MJ, Walford G, et al. Long-term outcomes of coronary-artery bypass grafting

versus stent implantation. N Engl J Med 2005; 352:2174–83.

[57] Tsuyuki RT, Shrive FM, Galbraith PD, et alfor the APPROACH Investigators. Revascularization in patients with heart failure. CMAJ 2006;175(4):361–5.

ELSEVIER
SAUNDERS

Heart Failure Clin 3 (2007) 229–235

HEART
FAILURE
CLINICS

Revascularization in Heart Failure: The Role of Percutaneous Coronary Intervention

Ajay J. Kirtane, MD, SM[a,b], Jeffrey W. Moses, MD[a,*]

[a]Columbia University Medical Center, New York, NY, USA
[b]Cardiovascular Research Foundation, New York, NY, USA

Ischemic heart disease is the leading cause of heart failure in North America, accounting for approximately two thirds of heart failure cases [1]. Patients who have ischemic heart failure suffer from higher rates of ischemic events, arrhythmic events, and increased mortality compared with patients who have normal ventricular function. Although there are inadequate clinical trial data in this patient population, coronary revascularization, either by way of percutaneous coronary intervention (PCI) or coronary artery bypass grafting (CABG), has the potential to provide relief of symptoms, improve ventricular performance, and possibly improve mortality in patients who have potentially revascularizable and viable myocardium [2–4]. Although the performance of coronary revascularization in patients who have depressed ventricular function is associated with a greater overall risk for adverse periprocedural events [5–7] compared with similar patients who have normal ventricular function, performance of PCI or CABG in this particular subset of patients may also be associated with the greatest absolute benefit afforded through revascularization [6,8].

Criteria for revascularization in heart failure patients

For a patient with heart failure to be considered a suitable candidate to truly benefit from coronary revascularization, ischemic heart disease should be at least a significant cause of the patient's depressed ventricular function and clinical heart failure. Although this statement may seem trite, its importance cannot be overstated. Because coronary artery disease is so common, patients who have cardiomyopathy of nonischemic origin frequently have coexistent and often incidental coronary artery disease. Such patients may derive some benefit from coronary revascularization, but the risks of PCI and CABG, including periprocedural adverse events and the requirement for long-term antiplatelet therapies, are not insignificant. The benefit of revascularization in such patients is not likely to be as great as for a patient who has cardiomyopathy wholly caused by ischemic coronary artery disease.

Several factors must be present for a patient who has ischemic cardiomyopathy to be considered a suitable candidate for improvement through revascularization. Patient-related factors include a reasonable life expectancy from other coexistent disease states and a relative paucity of other comorbidities (eg, chronic kidney disease, cerebrovascular disease, pulmonary disease, and so forth), particularly for patients being considered for CABG. In general, patients who are good revascularization candidates have a significant amount of demonstrably ischemic or hibernating (ie, viable) myocardium, or anginal symptoms [2,9,10]. Finally, the ischemic or hibernating territory should be amenable to revascularization either through PCI or CABG. For PCI, this implies lesions that can be treated with a percutaneous approach with the overall goal of maximal revascularization of ischemic or hibernating territories. In the case of CABG, this generally implies the presence of distal vasculature suitable for

* Corresponding author. Center for Interventional Vascular Therapy, Columbia University Medical Center and the Cardiovascular Research Foundation, New York, NY 10032.

  E-mail address: jmoses@crf.org (J.W. Moses).

1551-7136/07/$ - see front matter © 2007 Elsevier Inc. All rights reserved.
doi:10.1016/j.hfc.2007.05.003

heartfailure.theclinics.com

grafting (epicardial distal target with adequate runoff, adequate luminal size, absence of diffuse disease, and relative paucity of intervening stenoses that would limit potential backfilling from a bypass conduit).

Noninvasive methods of demonstrating the presence of ischemic or hibernating myocardium include exercise or pharmacologic stress testing with adjunctive perfusion or functional imaging. In our experience, standard exercise testing without imaging is of limited use in this population. Many patients who have heart failure and depressed ventricular function have abnormalities on the resting electrocardiogram that preclude accurate assessment of ischemic changes. Additionally, the goal of stress testing in this population is not solely to make the diagnosis of coronary artery disease but also to evaluate the amount of myocardium at risk to better form an appropriate revascularization strategy. Both of these factors limit the usefulness of traditional electrocardiography-based stress testing in the assessment of patients who have depressed ventricular function. The adjunctive use of imaging in conjunction with an exercise or pharmacologic stress study by way of either nuclear single photon emission computed tomography (SPECT) or echocardiography can be of great value in detecting ischemic myocardium in this patient population. Additionally, the use of positron emission tomography scanning, MRI, nuclear perfusion imaging with thallium redistribution, or dobutamine echocardiography can determine the presence of chronically ischemic or hibernating myocardium that is dysfunctional but nonetheless viable and may recover function following revascularization [9–12].

As a general rule, as the amount of myocardium at risk increases (eg, through a greater number of diseased vessels or more proximal vessel location) [13,14], the overall risks and absolute benefits of any revascularization strategy (PCI or CABG) increase over a strategy of medical therapy alone. It is the authors' opinion that most patients in the heart failure population who are reasonable candidates for revascularization and myocardium that is ischemic or hibernating should undergo some form of revascularization because of the prospect of improved left ventricular function. Nonetheless, given the relative paucity of data in this area, current guidelines are more guarded in their recommendations for revascularization in such patients, particularly those who do not have clinical angina [1].

Modes of revascularization in heart failure patients

The choice of PCI versus CABG in patients who have heart failure is a complex one that cannot be solely based on an algorithmic approach using the published literature as a guide. Although there have been many studies comparing PCI and CABG in patients who have ischemic heart disease, most of these studies have excluded patients who have heart failure or significant ventricular dysfunction [15–21], yielding limited randomized data regarding the preferred modality of revascularization in the heart failure population. Additionally, randomized trials of PCI versus CABG have been shown to be poorly representative of overall clinical practice, with one study demonstrating that only 36% of patients seen in routine clinical practice were eligible for participation in trials comparing PCI with CABG [22].

The randomized study that has specifically addressed the question of PCI versus CABG in patients ineligible for prior clinical studies (including those who had left ventricular dysfunction) was the AWESOME trial, a randomized comparison of PCI versus CABG in 554 patients enrolled at 16 Veterans Affairs Medical Centers [23]. In this trial overall survival was similar among patients randomized to PCI or CABG, and specifically in the subgroup of patients who had low ejection fractions (defined as <35%) 3-year survival was similar with both therapies (69% versus 72%, P not significant). Similarly, survival free of unstable angina or repeat revascularization was similar in both groups (37% with PCI versus 41% with CABG, P not significant) [24]. The study findings from the randomized cohort of patients in AWESOME were paralleled in the registry of patients who were eligible for the study but were not enrolled. Importantly, outcomes in the AWESOME registry did not differ between PCI and CABG among patients who received either therapy because of physician or patient preference, and PCI was more cost effective.

From a pragmatic standpoint, what the prior randomized PCI versus CABG trials and registry data (not just limited to patients who had heart failure or depressed ventricular function) have demonstrated consistently is that PCI is safe and effective, but is associated with a greater incidence of repeat revascularization compared with CABG [15,19,25,26], presumably because of the combination of restenosis and disease progression of nontreated lesions. The most marked benefit of CABG over PCI seems to be in the predictable and sustained patency of a left internal mammary artery (LIMA) bypass graft to the left anterior descending (LAD) coronary artery in patients who have left main or a proximal-mid left anterior descending coronary artery stenosis [27]. Many current interventionalists and surgeons largely base their recommendations regarding CABG versus PCI in patients in whom both are feasible on the following factors: (1) presence of a patent and usable LIMA conduit, (2) presence of severe stenosis in the left main coronary artery or the proximal LAD, and (3) LAD amenable to revascularization with the LIMA. If any of these three factors are not present, many consider CABG to provide less overall benefit compared with PCI. Conversely, if the LAD supplies a viable territory not amenable to PCI, CABG would be the preferred strategy.

Particularly among patients who have heart failure in whom the goal of revascularization is to preserve as much myocardial function as possible, an additional factor that would sway the balance in favor of CABG would be the ability to potentially perform more complete revascularization. The need for another surgical procedure (such as concomitant mitral or aortic valve surgery) could also sway a revascularization decision in favor of surgical revascularization, although initial data on a "hybrid" approach combining PCI with surgery for valvular disease has been promising [28], and this approach is being considered more frequently in the era of drug-eluting stents. Particular attention to comorbidities is also important when considering the roles of PCI or CABG; concomitant pulmonary, cerebrovascular, or renal disease can significantly increase the risks of performing CABG, particularly in patients who have ventricular dysfunction. Similarly, patients who have prior CABG may fare better with a strategy of PCI over repeat CABG [29].

Even if several factors that would historically seem to favor CABG over PCI in an individual patient are present, the impressive results of drug-eluting stenting in reducing restenosis and therefore target lesion revascularization [30,31] have begun to sway many interventionalists in favor of PCI as an initial revascularization strategy, particularly when dealing with focal coronary artery disease that is amenable to complete revascularization. Because most data comparing outcomes of patients treated with PCI versus CABG are derived from the balloon angioplasty era and early stenting experiences, these data do not address the revolutionary impact that drug-eluting stenting has had on the practice of revascularization for ischemic coronary artery disease. Many have hypothesized that drug-eluting stent technology has the potential to narrow the gap between CABG and PCI by limiting the rate of repeat revascularization among PCI-treated patients. This hypothesis is the subject of several ongoing studies, including ARTS-II, in which 3-year follow-up data demonstrated similar rates of mortality, myocardial infarction, and repeat revascularization among patients who had multivessel disease treated with drug-eluting stents compared with a similar cohort of CABG patients from ARTS-I (P. Serruys, unpublished data, 2006). Whether these initial results are sustained at longer follow-up, and additionally, whether these results are directly translatable to a heart failure population remains to be seen.

In summary, the ultimate goal of revascularization in patients who have heart failure is in maximizing the preservation of myocardial function. The choice of the optimal revascularization strategy in a given patient is based on an integrated assessment of patient-specific and anatomy-specific factors. New data comparing the use of drug-eluting stents to surgical revascularization is emerging and will help to better direct us regarding the most appropriate use of PCI or CABG. The remainder of this article is focused on the performance of PCI in patients who have heart failure.

Risks of revascularization and technical considerations in patients who have heart failure

Heart failure, either assessed clinically or measured through assessments of left ventricular performance, such as ejection fraction, has been shown to be independently associated with a greater risk for periprocedural complications among patients undergoing revascularization [5,7,32]. Optimization of patients' clinical status during PCI is thus necessary. Aside from a baseline assessment of ventricular function, it is critical to assess and actively manage the hemodynamic status of the patient before and during PCI. Patients who have elevated pulmonary capillary wedge pressure or acute pulmonary congestion may simply be unable to tolerate supine positioning for an extended period of time without antecedent diuresis or continuing respiratory support. Such patients may benefit from deferral of the procedure pending stabilization of respiratory status. If this is not possible, these patients may require aggressive sedation or semi-elective intubation to successfully undergo revascularization procedures.

Similarly, patients who have acutely worsening or fluctuating renal function may be less likely to tolerate significant amounts of intravenous contrast often necessary for effective percutaneous revascularization, and may also benefit from acute stabilization of renal status before revascularization or periprocedural ultrafiltration or hemodialysis to minimize long-term renal complications [33]. These patients may also benefit more from a staged approach to revascularization because total amount of contrast administered has been demonstrated to increase the risk for incident contrast-induced nephropathy following diagnostic and interventional coronary procedures [34]. Finally, actively ischemic patients are at higher risk for periprocedural complications, such as cardiogenic shock and mortality, because of diminished contractile reserve. Such patients may also benefit from a staged procedural approach of immediate stabilization and revascularization of the vessel subtending the actively ischemic or infarcting territory followed by urgent rather than emergent revascularization of other territories.

Many patients who have ischemic heart failure have severe coronary artery disease with technically challenging lesions, including diffusely diseased vessels, severely calcified arteries, bifurcation disease, left main coronary artery stenosis, saphenous vein graft disease from prior CABG, and chronic total occlusions (CTOs). As a result, PCI in these patients is often far more complex than in patients who have less severe coronary artery disease. These patients often require longer procedure times, greater amounts of contrast media, and the use of advanced PCI techniques and adjunctive devices. The use of atheroablative therapies necessary to deal with severe calcification, such as rotational atherectomy, for example, can lead to myocardial stunning because of distal microembolization of ablated plaque even if meticulous technique is used. This risk is of particular concern in patients who have depressed ventricular function who may not be able to tolerate further decrements in ventricular function. Similarly, patients who have heart failure and large territories at risk may not tolerate PCI-related complications, such as abrupt closure [13,14]. Patients who have degenerated saphenous vein grafts may poorly tolerate no-reflow caused by distal embolization of atherothrombotic debris, and thus consideration should be given to the use of embolic protection devices that reduce the rates

of adverse periprocedural events that seem related to emboli [35]. These patients may not be able to tolerate even the brief periods of occlusion that are required for the use of balloon-occlusion embolic protection devices, however, and not all patients are candidates for filter-based devices that preserve flow during the PCI.

Special concern should be paid to revascularization of chronic total occlusions, which are commonly observed in patients undergoing coronary angiography as a whole but are particularly prevalent among patients who have depressed ventricular function. Although chronic total occlusions are observed on more than 20% of diagnostic coronary angiograms in symptomatic patients [36,37], these lesions are infrequently attempted by PCI, partly because of the historically low overall success rates of PCI in this lesion subset [37,38]. Patients who have depressed ventricular function and viable myocardium have potentially the most to gain from revascularization of CTOs. One of the potential drawbacks of PCI versus CABG is an inability to achieve complete revascularization of ischemic territories; thus, if PCI is chosen as a strategy of revascularization, it behooves the operator to achieve as "CABG-like" a result as possible, and this includes attempted revascularization of CTOs. Despite the poorer results with CTO revascularization compared with other lesion subsets, successful revascularization of CTOs is possible with specialized and advanced techniques, with success rates greater than 80% in the hands of experienced operators [25,37,38]. In stable patients, PCI of occluded arteries is often attempted before PCI of other ischemic territories to minimize the ischemia that can occur during PCI of nonoccluded vessels by potentially reversing collateral flow in cases of abrupt or transient occlusion.

Need and use of support when performing percutaneous coronary intervention in patients who have heart failure

In patients who are clinically unstable or have high-risk lesions, various forms of hemodynamic and circulatory support have been used and proposed as adjunctive therapies to mitigate the risk associated with PCI in patients who have depressed ventricular function. Although there are limited data that can reproducibly identify the patients who would benefit most from hemodynamic support, patients who have severely depressed ejection fractions, cardiogenic shock, a large area of myocardium at risk, or a "last remaining vessel" seem to be at higher risk for hemodynamic compromise during PCI [39,40]. Nonetheless, the decision to use hemodynamic support during PCI is a patient-based decision that must weigh the potential benefit of these therapies against the not insignificant rate of complications with the use of these devices, some of which require large sheath sizes and are therefore associated with a higher rate of vascular complications than conventional PCI.

The most commonly used form of hemodynamic support is the intra-aortic balloon pump (IABP), typically placed by way of the femoral artery through an 8-French introducing sheath (or smaller access if placed in sheathless fashion). The beneficial hemodynamic effects of IABP result from an increase in perfusion pressure of the coronary arteries and cerebral circulation during balloon inflation followed by afterload reduction and augmented forward stroke volume following balloon deflation. Most high-risk patients in whom supported PCI is being considered can be treated with an IABP with good results despite a greater risk for vascular complications [40,41]. Partial cardiopulmonary bypass, or cardiopulmonary support (CPS), with or without the addition of a membrane oxygenator to the standard CPS circuit, has also been used to support high-risk PCI in patients who have depressed ventricular function. The rate of vascular complications is high with CPS as a result of the requirement for large cannulae (15–18 French). Patients requiring prolonged support may develop a systemic inflammatory state, including hemolytic anemia and disseminated intravascular coagulation. Nonetheless, in selected cases CPS has been demonstrated to be feasible with favorable results in nonrandomized series [42,43].

There are several new support devices under study and that have been proposed to facilitate safe performance of PCI in high-risk patients. The TandemHeart, which requires transseptal puncture for the placement of a left atrial cannula, is a percutaneous left ventricular assist device that is able to provide flow rates up to 5 L/min. This device has been used to assist high-risk PCI and in a preliminary randomized trial was demonstrated to improve hemodynamics compared with IABP without a difference in severe adverse events [44]. The Impella Recover device, another percutaneously implanted left ventricular assist device that is deployed retrograde across the aortic valve, has been shown in preliminary series to be feasible and safe for use in high-risk patients [45] and is currently under investigation in a larger-scale trial.

Summary

The overall goal of revascularization in patients who have heart failure and left ventricular function is to try to improve symptoms, to prevent the occurrence of future ischemic or arrhythmic events, and to potentially improve ventricular function. The choice of a revascularization strategy must be based on the patient's baseline clinical status and presentation and a careful assessment of the risks and benefits of performing revascularization in the individual patient with particular attention to technical factors and the potential for complete revascularization. Carefully conducted studies and clinical trials are necessary to further determine the most appropriate revascularization strategy in this subgroup of patients. If PCI is chosen, it must be performed by experienced operators who have optimized the patient's clinical status and can perform PCI with a high likelihood of procedural and clinical success, and who are comfortable with several means of cardiac support. Irrespective of which revascularization strategy (PCI or CABG) is chosen, cross-consultation and open discussions between the treating interventionalist, surgeon, and cardiologist are necessary to ensure the most thoughtful and appropriate care for the patient.

References

[1] Hunt SA, Abraham WT, Chin MH, et al. ACC/AHA 2005 guideline update for the diagnosis and management of chronic heart failure in the adult: a report of the American College of Cardiology/American Heart Association Task Force on Practice Guidelines (Writing Committee to Update the 2001 Guidelines for the Evaluation and Management of Heart Failure). American College of Cardiology Web Site. Available at: http://www.acc.org/clinical/guidelines/failure/index.pdf. Accessed December 4, 2006.

[2] Allman KC, Shaw LJ, Hachamovitch R, et al. Myocardial viability testing and impact of revascularization on prognosis in patients with coronary artery disease and left ventricular dysfunction: a meta-analysis. J Am Coll Cardiol 2002;39:1151–8.

[3] Elefteriades JA, Tolis G Jr, Levi E, et al. Coronary artery bypass grafting in severe left ventricular dysfunction: excellent survival with improved ejection fraction and functional state. J Am Coll Cardiol 1993;22:1411–7.

[4] Baker DW, Jones R, Hodges J, et al. Management of heart failure. III. The role of revascularization in the treatment of patients with moderate or severe left ventricular systolic dysfunction. JAMA 1994;272: 1528–34.

[5] Holmes DR, Selzer F, Johnston JM, et al. Modeling and risk prediction in the current era of interventional cardiology: a report from the National Heart, Lung, and Blood Institute Dynamic Registry. Circulation 2003;107:1871–6.

[6] Alderman EL, Fisher LD, Litwin P, et al. Results of coronary artery surgery in patients with poor left ventricular function (CASS). Circulation 1983;68: 785–95.

[7] Keelan PC, Johnston JM, Koru-Sengul T, et al. Comparison of in-hospital and one-year outcomes in patients with left ventricular ejection fractions ≤40%, 41% to 49%, and ≥50% having percutaneous coronary revascularization. Am J C ardiol 2003; 91:1168–72.

[8] Passamani E, Davis KB, Gillespie MJ, et al. A randomized trial of coronary artery bypass surgery. Survival of patients with a low ejection fraction. N Engl J Med 1985;312:1665–71.

[9] Pagano D, Bonser RS, Townend JN, et al. Predictive value of dobutamine echocardiography and positron emission tomography in identifying hibernating myocardium in patients with postischaemic heart failure. Heart 1998;79:281–8.

[10] Di Carli MF, Asgarzadie F, Schelbert HR, et al. Quantitative relation between myocardial viability and improvement in heart failure symptoms after revascularization in patients with ischemic cardiomyopathy. Circulation 1995;92:3436–44.

[11] Kim RJ, Wu E, Rafael A, et al. The use of contrast-enhanced magnetic resonance imaging to identify reversible myocardial dysfunction. N Engl J Med 2000;343:1445–53.

[12] Kim RJ, Manning WJ. Viability assessment by delayed enhancement cardiovascular magnetic resonance: will low-dose dobutamine dull the shine? Circulation 2004;109:2476–9.

[13] Ellis SG, Myler RK, King SB 3rd, et al. Causes and correlates of death after unsupported coronary angioplasty: implications for use of angioplasty and advanced support techniques in high-risk settings. Am J Cardiol 1991;68:1447–51.

[14] Califf RM, Phillips HR 3rd, Hindman MC, et al. Prognostic value of a coronary artery jeopardy score. J Am Coll Cardiol 1985;5:1055–63.

[15] The Bypass Angioplasty Revascularization Investigation (BARI) Investigators. Comparison of coronary bypass surgery with angioplasty in patients with multivessel disease. N Engl J Med 1996;335: 217–25.

[16] Serruys PW, Unger F, Sousa JE, et al. Comparison of coronary-artery bypass surgery and stenting for the treatment of multivessel disease. N Engl J Med 2001;344:1117–24.

[17] Srinivas VS, Brooks MM, Detre KM, et al. Contemporary percutaneous coronary intervention versus balloon angioplasty for multivessel coronary artery disease: a comparison of the National Heart, Lung and Blood Institute Dynamic Registry and the Bypass Angioplasty Revascularization Investigation (BARI) Study. Circulation 2002;106:1627–33.

[18] Rodriguez A, Bernardi V, Navia J, et al. Argentine randomized study: coronary angioplasty with stenting versus coronary bypass surgery in patients with multiple-vessel disease (ERACI II): 30-day and one-year follow-up results. J Am Coll Cardiol 2001;37:51–8.

[19] Pocock SJ, Henderson RA, Rickards AF, et al. Meta-analysis of randomised trials comparing coronary angioplasty with bypass surgery. Lancet 1995; 346:1184–9.

[20] King SB, Lembo NJ, Weintraub WS, et al. A randomized trial comparing coronary angioplasty with coronary bypass surgery. N Engl J Med 1994;331: 1044–50.

[21] CABRI trial participants. First-year results of CABRI (Coronary Angioplasty versus Bypass Revascularisation Investigation). Lancet 1995;346:1179–84.

[22] Hordijk-Trion M, Lenzen M, Wijns W, et al. Patients enrolled in coronary intervention trials are not representative of patients in clinical practice: results from the Euro Heart Survey on Coronary Revascularization. Eur Heart J 2006;27:671–8.

[23] Morrison DA, Sethi G, Sacks J, et al. Percutaneous coronary intervention versus coronary bypass graft surgery for patients with medically refractory myocardial ischemia and risk factors for adverse outcomes with bypass: the VA AWESOME multicenter registry: comparison with the randomized clinical trial. J Am Coll Cardiol 2002;39:266–73.

[24] Sedlis SP, Ramanathan KB, Morrison DA, et al. Outcome of percutaneous coronary intervention versus coronary bypass grafting for patients with low left ventricular ejection fractions, unstable angina pectoris, and risk factors for adverse outcomes with bypass (the AWESOME Randomized Trial and Registry). Am J Cardiol 2004;94: 118–20.

[25] Stone GW, Reifart NJ, Moussa I, et al. Percutaneous recanalization of chronically occluded coronary arteries: a consensus document: part II. Circulation 2005;112:2530–7.

[26] Mercado N, Wijns W, Serruys PW, et al. One-year outcomes of coronary artery bypass graft surgery versus percutaneous coronary intervention with multiple stenting for multisystem disease: a meta-analysis of individual patient data from randomized clinical trials. J Thorac Cardiovasc Surg 2005;130: 512–9.

[27] Gibbons RJ, Abrams J, Chatterjee K, et al. ACC/ AHA 2002 guideline update for the management of patients with chronic stable angina: a report of the American College of Cardiology/American

Heart Association Task Force on Practice Guide-lines (Committee to Update the 1999 Guidelines for the Management of Patients with Chronic Stable Angina). Available at: www.acc.org/clinical/guidelines/stable/stable.pdf. Accessed December 4, 2006.

[28] Byrne JG, Leacche M, Unic D, et al. Staged initial percutaneous coronary intervention followed by valve surgery ("hybrid approach") for patients with complex coronary and valve disease. J Am Coll Cardiol 2005;45:14–8.

[29] Morrison DA, Sethi G, Sacks J, et al. Percutaneous coronary intervention versus repeat bypass surgery for patients with medically refractory myocardial ischemia: AWESOME randomized trial and registry experience with post-CABG patients. J Am Coll Cardiol 2002;40:1951–4.

[30] Moses JW, Leon MB, Popma JJ, et al. Sirolimus-eluting stents versus standard stents in patients with stenosis in a native coronary artery. N Engl J Med 2003;349:1315–23.

[31] Stone GW, Ellis SG, Cox DA, et al. A polymer-based, paclitaxel-eluting stent in patients with coronary artery disease. N Engl J Med 2004;350:221–31.

[32] Anderson RD, Ohman EM, Holmes DR Jr, et al. Prognostic value of congestive heart failure history in patients undergoing percutaneous coronary interventions. J Am Coll Cardiol 1998;32:936–41.

[33] Marenzi G, Marana I, Lauri G, et al. The prevention of radiocontrast-agent-induced nephropathy by hemofiltration. N Engl J Med 2003;349:1333–40.

[34] Mehran R, Aymong ED, Nikolsky E, et al. A simple risk score for prediction of contrast-induced nephropathy after percutaneous coronary intervention: development and initial validation. J Am Coll Cardiol 2004;44:1393–9.

[35] Baim DS, Wahr D, George B, et al. Randomized trial of a distal embolic protection device during percutaneous intervention of saphenous vein aorto-coronary bypass grafts. Circulation 2002;105:1285–90.

[36] Kahn JK. Angiographic suitability for catheter revascularization of total coronary occlusions in patients from a community hospital setting. Am Heart J 1993;126:561–4.

[37] Stone GW, Kandzari DE, Mehran R, et al. Percutaneous recanalization of chronically occluded coronary arteries: a consensus document: part I. Circulation 2005;112:2364–72.

[38] Stone GW, Colombo A, Teirstein PS, et al. Percutaneous recanalization of chronically occluded coronary arteries: procedural techniques, devices, and results. Catheter Cardiovasc Interv 2005;66:217–36.

[39] Bergelson BA, Jacobs AK, Cupples LA, et al. Prediction of risk for hemodynamic compromise during percutaneous transluminal coronary angioplasty. Am J Cardiol 1992;70:1540–5.

[40] Smith SC Jr, Feldman TE, Hirshfeld JW Jr, et al. ACC/AHA/SCAI 2005 guideline update for percutaneous coronary intervention: a report of the American College of Cardiology/American Heart Association Task Force on Practice Guidelines (ACC/AHA/SCAI Writing Committee to Update the 2001 Guidelines for Percutaneous Coronary Intervention). American College of Cardiology Web Site. Available at: http://www.acc.org/clinical/guidelines/percutaneous/update/index.pdf. Accessed December 4, 2006.

[41] Kahn JK, Rutherford BD, McConahay DR, et al. Supported "high risk" coronary angioplasty using intraaortic balloon pump counterpulsation. J Am Coll Cardiol 1990;15:1151–5.

[42] Vogel RA, Shawl F, Tommaso C, et al. Initial report of the National registry of elective cardiopulmonary bypass supported coronary angioplasty. J Am Coll Cardiol 1990;15:23–9.

[43] Shawl FA, Quyyumi AA, Bajaj S, et al. Percutaneous cardiopulmonary bypass-supported coronary angioplasty in patients with unstable angina pectoris or myocardial infarction and a left ventricular ejection fraction ≤ 25%. Am J Cardiol 1996;77:14–9.

[44] Burkhoff D, Cohen H, Brunckhorst C, et al. A randomized multicenter clinical study to evaluate the safety and efficacy of the TandemHeart percutaneous ventricular assist device versus conventional therapy with intraaortic balloon pumping for treatment of cardiogenic shock. Am Heart J 2006;152:469. e1–8.

[45] Henriques JPS, Remmelink M, Baan JJ, et al. Safety and feasibility of elective high-risk percutaneous coronary intervention procedures with left ventricular support of the Impella recover LP 2.5. Am J Cardiol 2006;97:990–2.

ELSEVIER
SAUNDERS

Heart Failure Clin 3 (2007) 237–243

HEART
FAILURE
CLINICS

Left Ventricular Restoration: How Important is the Surgical Treatment of Ischemic Heart Failure Trial?

Lorenzo Menicanti, MD[a],*, Marisa Di Donato, MD[b]

[a]San Donato Hospital, San Donato Milanese, Milano, Italy
[b]University of Florence, Firenze, Italy

Chronic ischemic heart failure (CHF) is one of the major health care issues in the western world partly because of an aging population and more effective treatment of acute myocardial infarction [1,2]. Intensive medical management reduces symptoms and improves survival in CHF but patients in high functional classes (NYHA III-IV) still have a poor 3-year prognosis despite improved medical therapy, with high social and economic impact [3].

The increase in left ventricular (LV) volume following myocardial infarction (MI) is a component of the remodeling process characterized by LV volume increase and geometry abnormalities with frequently associated mitral regurgitation that leads to heart failure (HF) progression; this progression is independent of the neurohormonal activation, according to the biomechanical model of HF recently introduced by Mann and Bristow [4]. The concept of a biomechanical model of HF reinforces the need for therapies able to reduce LV volumes and restore geometry; the model also emphasizes the need for measuring LV volumes and geometric parameters and the importance of assessing the presence and the degree of mitral regurgitation in patients who have ischemic dilated cardiomyopathy and cardiac dysfunction.

Left ventricular shape and function abnormalities following myocardial infarction

A strict relationship exists between the shape of the LV and its function. The ellipsoid is the geometric form that most resembles the shape of the normal ventricle. It derives from the architecture of the anatomic distribution of cardiac muscle fibers. The double spiral that constitutes the three-dimensional (3-D) architecture of the heart permits a shortening of 15% of the fibers to give an ejection fraction of 60% and the different distribution of the fibers within the wall from the epicardium to the endocardium accounts for the twisting effect of the apex that optimizes the ejection of blood into the aortic vessel. The elliptic shape enhances blood flow at the inflow and outflow tract. When disease alters the shape of the ventricle, the equilibrium of forces and of spatial orientation of the fibers in the LV is altered and loses its optimal function. The extracellular matrix (cardiac interstitium and collagen) markedly contributes to connect the myocytes in a complex array of fibers forming the 3-D architecture of the wall and coordinating the delivery of forces generated by myocytes. These forces are important determinants of diastolic and systolic stiffness and serve to resist deformation, maintain shape and wall thickness, and prevent ventricular bulging and rupture [5].

Shape changes after MI (especially if anterior) mainly consist of a reduction of curvature radius (the reciprocal of internal radius) at the apical level that creates a high local tension. The increase in tension plays a key role in activating complex neurohormonal mechanisms, including an increase in angiotensin II, collagen deposition, and degradation through metalloproteinase-1 and -2 activation. This activation may induce apoptosis launching the complex process called remodeling, which characterizes ischemic cardiomyopathy [5–8]. The increase in chamber volume

---

* Corresponding author. Department of Cardiac Surgery, San Donato Hospital, Via Morandi 30, 20097 San Donato Milanese, Milano, Italy.

E-mail address: menicanti@libero.it (L. Menicanti).

doi:10.1016/j.hfc.2007.04.009

heartfailure.theclinics.com

compensates for the decreased performance of the ischemic or necrotic regions, thus increasing wall tension with a nonuniform distribution within the chamber that further dilates the ventricle. Frequently, the enlargement of the cavity is first an elongation of the major axis, which allows an elliptic shape (ie, an optimal or suboptimal short-to-long axis ratio). As the process continues, however, the short axis markedly dilates, the ratio between the two axes approaches one (sphere), and this leads to mitral valve incompetence.

The increase in the curvature radius induces an increase in parietal tension with changes in its regional temporal distribution attributable to myocardial structural etherogeneity. This process is responsible for the so-called "nonischemic expansion" that can involve also the basal portions of the ventricle leading to a global depression of LV pump function [6]. This case differs from the classic aneurysm, characterized by a dyskinetic portion of the ventricle demarcated by a neck that separates scarred from sound tissue. This type of lesion is no longer or rarely seen after MI now because of the early reperfusion that often leaves the scar only at the subendocardium.

Myocardial regional or global dysfunction can persist after successful early reperfusion leading to adverse remodeling and clinical HF in a consistent number of patients. Bolognese and colleagues [9] observed that in 30% of patients successfully treated with primary percutaneous transluminal coronary angioplasty, LV dilatation (defined as >20% increase in end-diastolic volume) is present 6 months after the procedure. Cardiac death and combined events rates were significantly higher among patients who had LV dilatation than among those who did not [9]. Treating the culprit lesion of acute MI with early revascularization thus may not be sufficient to guarantee the cure of that patient and it is necessary to check for the volume and the function of the ventricle to assess prognosis.

Mitral regurgitation (MR) is a common manifestation of dilated ischemic cardiomyopathy and its mechanism is linked to either an increased mitral annulus or a restrictive pattern of the posterior leaflet, which is pulled toward the apex during systole owing to papillary muscle lateral displacement (tethering). It has been reported that these mechanisms are determinants of functional MR in left ventricular remodeling [10] and we reported that regional inferior shape abnormality can also be a determinant [11]. In fact, in analyzing the wall curvature in a series of patients who

had chronic ischemic cardiomyopathy attributable to anterior infarction, patients who had MR showed a flattening of the inferior curvature that was significantly different from those of patients who had previous anterior MI without MR. Regional shape abnormalities were strictly related to inferior wall motion abnormalities in that inferior hypokinesia was detected in patients who had MR and not in patients who did not have MR. Fig. 1 reports geometric abnormalities detected in a series of patients who did and did not have MR. Fig. 2 shows geometric abnormalities according to the degree of MR. These data show that even a mild degree of MR is associated with significant geometric abnormalities.

The rationale to reshape

From what is reported above, it is clear that postinfarction ischemic cardiomyopathy is characterized by a markedly abnormal regional or global shape and function linked to each other in a vicious cycle that ultimately leads to the failing ventricle and to the clinical manifestation of heart failure. In light of the biomechanical model of heart failure, the great challenge should be to find a therapeutic strategy that may improve the function and the shape of the ventricle by reverting, arresting, or at least delaying the adverse remodeling process. Pharmacologic treatment with agents, such as angiotensin-converting enzyme inhibitors and beta-blockers, have been shown to be effective in improving functional status and survival [12]; these drugs can also induce a small reduction of volume but they do not change LV shape. Coronary artery bypass grafting (CABG) alone and mitral repair alone or in combination with CABG are also therapeutic strategies in ischemic dilated cardiomyopathy, but again their effect on sphericity and shape is irrelevant.

Surgical ventricular restoration for ischemic heart failure

Surgical ventricular restoration (SVR) introduced by Dor in 1985 [13] as a modification of the Cooley and Jatene [14,15] technique is one of the strategies that has the objective of reshaping the ventricle. Initially it was applied to the classic aneurysm following anterior MI; however, later Dor and coworkers [16] demonstrated that the procedure is also safe and effective in dilated ischemic cardiomyopathy (dyskinetic or akinetic

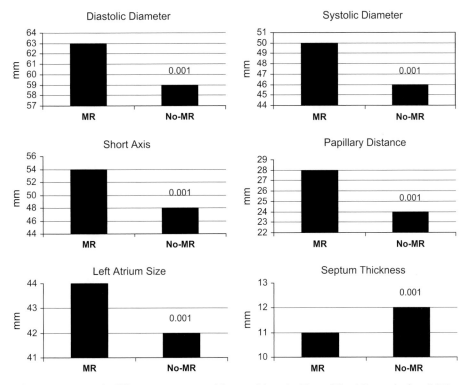

Fig. 1. LV geometric differences are reported in pts with and without Mitral Regurgitation (MR).

lesion). This finding was considered a step forward in the concept of surgical treatment of ischemic heart failure. In fact, the procedure tends to reorganize fiber architecture by circularly reducing the LV cavity. The exclusion of the necrotic tissue and the consequent reduction of volume lead to a reduction of parietal stress and a consequent improvement in regional wall motion.

SVR is considered a surgical alternative option for the treatment of ischemic heart disease when MI leaves regional asynergy, which determines dilatation and dysfunction of the LV. Observational results have shown that the technique is safe and effective in improving LV pump function, functional status, and survival [17–19]. The term SVR is often considered a synonym of aneurysmectomy, which creates some confusion in interpreting the results and in patient selection; aneurysmectomy approaches the classic aneurysm (ie, dyskinetic lesions), whereas SVR applies also to akinetic lesions. We have demonstrated that surgical outcome in a large series of patients treated with SVR is linked to the extent of asynergy rather than to the type (akinetic versus dyskinetic) [20].

This observation has helped to advance the belief that remodeling operation may be applied as surgical treatment in postinfarction dilated cardiomyopathy.

Past reports clarified why larger ventricular volumes might limit prognosis; Di Donato and coworkers [19] reported longitudinal survival studies that demonstrate better survival and functional outcome after SVR interventions when left ventricular end systolic volume index is not markedly increased. Athanasuleas and associates [17] reported similar late findings, especially in the recent 5-year follow-up of 1198 patients undergoing SVR in the recent RESTORE team report.

Need for a randomized trial

The ongoing Surgical Treatment of Ischemic Heart Failure (STICH) trial is an international, randomized, controlled clinical trial still in the recruitment phase that is testing the primary hypothesis (hypothesis 1) that CABG confers long-term mortality, morbidity, quality of life, or cost benefits over state-of-the art medical therapy in patients who have depressed ejection fraction (EF) ($\leq 35\%$) and coronary vessels amenable for grafting. The recruitment into the hypothesis 2 trial, testing whether surgical LV shape and size

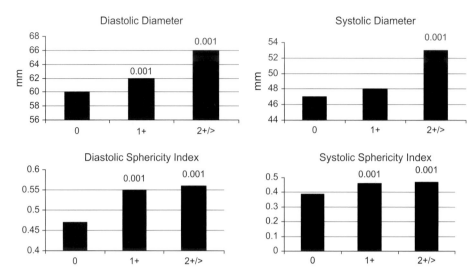

Fig. 2. LV dimensions and Sphericity index by the degree of mitral regurgitation are reported.

optimization by surgical ventricular restoration combined with CABG improves survival and morbidity and quality of life over CABG alone, was completed in January 2006, and the study is currently in the follow-up stage. To date, 2212 patients have been enrolled at 99 centers in 25 countries. Important secondary endpoints include morbidity, economics, and quality of life. Core laboratories for cardiac magnetic resonance, echocardiography, neurohormonal/cytokine/genetic, and radionuclide studies will ensure consistent testing practices and standardization of data necessary to identify eligible patients and to address specific questions related to the primary hypotheses.

Two other important substudies are part of the STICH trial: (1) the study of Dobutamine Echocardiography in Patients with Ischemic Heart Failure Evaluated for Revascularization (DECI-PHER-STICH), that will test whether coronary revascularization improves 3-year survival over medical therapy in patients who have myocardial viability demonstrated by dobutamine echocardiography versus those who do not have myocardial viability, and (2) the study of Mitral Regurgitation Transesophageal Echocardiography (MR TEE) that will address the mechanisms, prognosis, and impact of STICH interventions on functional mitral regurgitation in ischemic cardiomyopathy using transesophageal echocardiography (TEE).

The need for this randomized trial for both hypotheses is because (1) data on the superiority of surgery in respect to medical therapy are old and obtained in small series of patients from the CASS study that analyzed few patients who had a depressed EF [21] and (2) data on the effectiveness of adding SVR to CABG are observational and need to be validated.

Despite a lack of evidence proving the superiority of one strategy over all others, cardiologists and surgeons secretly—or not so secretly—believe they know the best way to care for their patients. Some investigators are hesitant to randomize because they believe that all patients should have bypass surgery and others believe that none of these patients should have surgery. This difference of opinion occurs within the same country and sometimes within the same city. On both sides, people are equally convinced that they are right. In reality, large numbers of patients fall into a gray zone without clear evidence for benefit from medical treatment, CABG, or CABG and SVR [22].

STICH is the most important randomized medical-surgical trial after CASS in the treatment of coronary artery disease.

Expectations from the Surgical Treatment of Ischemic Heart Failure Trial: surgical arm, hypothesis 2

The surgical arm includes patients who have ongoing refractory angina or left main/equivalent critical stenosis who will receive CABG alone or

CABG plus SVR. Hypothesis 2 (surgical arm) tests whether surgical LV shape and size optimization by SVR combined with CABG improves survival, morbidity, and quality of life over CABG alone. Patients in this arm should have LV characteristics amenable for SVR (ie, volume enlargement, a certain extent of asynergy in the anterior region, and potentially recoverable remote, nonscarred segments).

Besides the primary hypothesis, the trial will answer relevant clinical questions; first, it will focus on the recognition of the potentially lethal complications of enlarging ventricular volume after myocardial infarction. This fundamental concept stems from the work of White and colleagues [23], showing how increased left ventricular end-systolic volume affects mortality. The congestive heart failure community recognizes that measuring LV volumes with any imaging method (angiography, echocardiography, nuclear imaging studies, cardiac magnetic resonance) is an important measurement that reflects a major change from conventional analysis because ejection fraction is now the accepted, traditional prognostic indicator. Nonrandomized studies [24] in which the entry criterion was LVESVI of approximately 60 mL/m^2 that compared medical therapy and CABG demonstrated that prognosis was determined by LVESVI changes over 4 years and was independent of the treatment category.

Second, an important concept that the STICH trial will address is the potential recovery of function of remote nonscarred regions after the scar is excluded by SVR; we will learn by means of magnetic resonance imaging, ventriculography, echocardiography, and nuclear medicine studies of remote regions if there is sufficient compensatory muscle to resume function. As for the primary hypothesis of restoration, the trial will definitively demonstrate whether the reduction of volume induced by SVR and the surgical exclusion of the scar associated with CABG will add benefits to patients who have dilated ischemic cardiomyopathy and heart failure.

Several studies demonstrated that the exclusion of the scar improves tissue homogeneity in contiguous segments, thus improving contraction and relaxation synchrony [25–27]; from the STICH trial we will know the rate of biventricular pacing implantation in SVR patients in respect to treatment with CABG alone. Another important issue concerns ventricular arrhythmias and the rate of sudden death in the STICH population.

Our data and those from other studies [28–33] show that ventricular arrhythmias are significantly reduced by SVR and that the rate of sudden death is low in patients treated with this procedure. The Multicenter Automatic Defibrillator Implantation Trial (MADIT) and MADIT II [34,35] and recent results presented at the American Heart Association (AHA) 2006 meeting in Chicago show that heart failure remains the leading cause of death for patients who have implanted defibrillator (ICD); they are at increased risk for heart failure and non–sudden cardiac death and most of them still ultimately die uncomfortable, slow deaths from heart failure. In the EVADEF registry, Le Heuzey and colleagues [36] tracked 2418 patients implanted with an ICD for various underlying causes at 22 centers in France between 2001 and 2003, with follow-up to 2005. There were 274 deaths, 115 (37.5%) of which were from heart failure and 24 (13%) of which were from cardiac arrest with electromechanical dissociation. Other causes included fatal arrhythmias (6%), cancer (11%), septic shock (6.9%), and complications from heart transplant procedures (4.6%). Stewart and Stevenson [37,38] from Brigham and Women's Hospital have developed a way to discuss the issue with patients: "We tell them that of 100 patients who receive an ICD, 30 will die anyway in the next five years, seven or eight will be saved by the device, 10 to 20 will receive inappropriate shocks that are painful and debilitating, and five to 15 will suffer complications besides unnecessary shocks."

Overall, from these recent AHA discussion the presenters [37] agreed that the "benefit of ICDs is not as big as we think." We do believe that ICD treats the electrical causes of the disease and that SVR treats the underlying disease (ie, LV dilatation with increased stress and stretch, scar ventricular arrhythmias triggering, inhomogeneity of myocardial tissue, and myocardial ischemia). All these factors are corrected by SVR: stress, stretch and volume reduction, scar exclusion, and ischemia relief. Although the STICH trial does not specifically address ventricular arrhythmias or resynchronization therapy (RCT) therapy, we will have the opportunity to know the incidence of RCT-ICD implantation in the three arms, the rate of sudden death, and the frequency of appropriate firings. To address these questions, however, we should wait until the end of follow-up of the STICH patients, which will be approximately at the end of 2010.

Summary

If the two primary hypotheses of the STICH trial are demonstrated and surgical therapy is proved to be superior to medical therapy, early aggressive evaluation of coronary artery disease as a potentially correctable cause of new-onset HF would be the preferred strategy. This strategy could tremendously change the treatment of ischemic heart disease. Confirming the STICH revascularization hypothesis will dramatically increase the use of CABG among the millions of patients now being medically treated without evaluation for an ischemic cause. SVR is not a standardized procedure and different surgical techniques can be applied in the STICH population; moreover, surgical experience may favor the beneficial effects of SVR and we hope that the trial will focus also on the role of experience and of technical differences to avoid unbiased results.

References

[1] Califf RM, Adams KF, McKenna WJ, et al. A randomized controlled trial of epoprostenol therapy for severe congestive heart failure: the Flolan international randomized survival trial. (FIRST). Am Heart J 1997;134:44–54.

[2] Greenberg B, Quinones MA, Koilpillai C, et al. Effects of long-term enalapril therapy on cardiac structure and function in patients with left ventricular dysfunction. Circulation 1995;91:2573–81.

[3] Watson RDS, Gibbs CR, Lip GY. ABC of heart failure: clinical features and complications. BMJ 2000; 320:236–9.

[4] Mann DL, Bristow MR. Mechanisms and models in heart failure. The biochemical model and beyond. Circulation 2005;111:2837–49.

[5] Weber KT. Cardiac interstitium in health and disease: the fibrillar collagen network. J Am Coll Cardiol 1989;13:1637–52.

[6] Bogaert J, Bosmans H, Maes A, et al. Remote myocardial dysfunction after acute anterior myocardial infarction: impact of left ventricular shape on regional function: a magnetic resonance myocardial tagging study. J Am Coll Cardiol 2000;35:1525–34.

[7] Dorn GW 2nd. Adrenergic pathways and left ventricular remodeling. J Card Fail 2002;8(6 Suppl): S370–3.

[8] Peterson JT, Hallak H, Johnson L, et al. Matrix metalloproteinase inhibition attenuates left ventricular remodeling and dysfunction in a rat model of progressive heart failure. Circulation 2001;103:2303–9.

[9] Bolognese L, Carrabba N, Parodi G, et al. Impact of microvascular dysfunction on left ventricular remodeling and long-term clinical outcome after primary coronary angioplasty for acute myocardial infarction. Circulation 2004;109(9):1121–6.

[10] Yiu SF, Enriquez-Sarano M, Tribouilloy C, et al. Determinants of the degree of functional mitral regurgitation in patients with systolic left ventricular dysfunction: a quantitative clinical study. Circulation 2000;102:1400–6.

[11] Toso A, Sabatier M, Dor V, et al. Regional curvature and wall motion abnormalities in anterior post-infarction cardiomyopathy with functional mitral regurgitation. Eur Heart J 2002;23(S):716.

[12] Packer M, Bristow MR, Cohn JN, et al. The effect of carvedilol on morbidity and mortality in patients with chronic heart failure. U.S. Carvedilol Heart Failure Study Group. N Engl J Med 1996;334: 1349–55.

[13] Dor V, Kreitmann P, Jourdan J, et al. Interest of physiological closure (circumferential plasty on contractile areas) of left ventricle after resection and endocardectomy for aneurysm of akinetic zone: comparison with classical technique about a series of 209 left ventricular resections. J Card Surg 1985; 26:73.

[14] Cooley D. Ventricular endoaneurysmorrhaphy: a simplified repair for extensive postinfarction aneurysm. J Card Surg 1989;4:200–5.

[15] Jatene AD. Left ventricular aneurysmectomy: resection or reconstruction. J Thorac Cardiovasc Surg 1985;89:321–31.

[16] Dor V, Sabatier M, Di Donato M, et al. Late hemodynamic results after left ventricular patch repair associated with coronary grafting in patients with postinfarction akinetic or dyskinetic aneurysm of the left ventricle. J Thorac Cardiovasc Surg 1995; 110:1291–301.

[17] Athanasuleas CL, Buckberg GD, Stanley AWH, et al. Surgical ventricular restoration in the treatment of congestive heart failure due to post-infarction ventricular dilation. J Am Coll Cardiol 2004; 44:1439–45.

[18] Menicanti L, Di Donato M. The Dor procedure: what has changed after fifteen years of clinical practice? J Thorac Cardiovasc Surg 2002;124:886–90.

[19] Di Donato M, Toso A, Maioli M, et al. Intermediate survival and predictors of death after surgical ventricular restoration. Semin Thorac Cardiovasc Surg 2001;13(4):468–75.

[20] Di Donato M, Sabatier M, Dor V, et al. Akinetic versus dyskinetic postinfarction scar: relation to surgical outcome in patients undergoing endoventricular circular patch plasty repair. J Am Coll Cardiol 1997;29:1569–75.

[21] Killip T, Passamani E, Davis K. Coronary artery surgery study (CASS): a randomized trial of coronary bypass surgery. Eight years follow-up and survival in patients with reduced ejection fraction. Circulation 1985;72(6 Pt 2):V102–9.

[22] Doenst T, Velazquez EJ, Beyersdorf F, et al. STICH investigators. To STICH or not to STICH:

we know the answer, but do we understand the question? J Thorac Cardiovasc Surg 2005;129(2): 246–9.

[23] White HD, Norris RM, Brown MA, et al. Left ventricular end-systolic volume as the major determinant of survival after recovery from myocardial infarction. Circulation 1987;76:44–51.

[24] Senior R, Lahiri A, Kaul S. Effect of revascularization on left ventricular remodeling in patients with heart failure from severe chronic ischemic left ventricular dysfunction. Am J Cardiol 2001;88:624–9 54(Suppl III):III107–17.

[25] Di Donato M, Toso A, Dor V, et al. RESTORE Group. Surgical ventricular restoration improves mechanical intraventricular dyssynchrony in ischemic cardiomyopathy. Circulation 2004;109(21): 2536–43.

[26] Tulner SA, Steendijk P, Klautz RJ, et al. Surgical ventricular restoration in patients with ischemic dilated cardiomyopathy: evaluation of systolic and diastolic ventricular function, wall stress, dyssynchrony, and mechanical efficiency by pressure-volume loops. J Thorac Cardiovasc Surg 2006; 132(3):610–20.

[27] Schreuder JJ, Castiglioni A, Maisano F, et al. Acute decrease of left ventricular mechanical dyssynchrony and improvement of contractile state and energy efficiency after left ventricular restoration. J Thorac Cardiovasc Surg 2005;129(1):138–45.

[28] Di Donato M, Sabatier M, Dor V, RESTORE Group. Surgical ventricular restoration in patients with postinfarction coronary artery disease: effectiveness on spontaneous and inducible ventricular tachycardia. Semin Thorac Cardiovasc Surg 2001; 13(4):480–5.

[29] Di Donato M, Sabatier M, Dor V, et al. RESTORE Group. Ventricular arrhythmias after LV remodelling: surgical ventricular restoration or ICD? Heart Fail Rev 2004;9(4):299–306.

[30] Mickleborough LL, Merchant N, Ivanov J, et al. Left ventricular reconstruction: early and late results. J Thorac Cardiovasc Surg 2004;128(1):27–37.

[31] Dor V, Sabatier M, Montiglio F, et al. Results of non guided subtotal endicardiectomy associated with left ventricular reconstruction in patients with ischemic ventricular arrhythmias. J Thorac Cardiovasc Surg 1994;197:1301–7.

[32] Dor V. The treatment of refractory ischemic ventricular tachycardia by endo-ventricular patch plasty reconstruction of the left ventricle. Semin Thorac Cardiovasc Surg 1997;9(2):146–55.

[33] Sosa E, Scanavacca M, d'Avila A, et al. Long-term results of visually guided left ventricular reconstruction single therapy to treat ventricular tachycardia associated with post-infarction anteroseptal aneurysm. J Cardiovasc Elecytrophysiol 1998;9:1133–43.

[34] Moss AJ, Greeberg H, Case RB, et al. Elkin AD for the Multicenter Automatic Defibrillator Implantation Trial-II (MADIT-II) Research Group. Long term clinical course of patients after termination of ventricular tachyarrhythmias by an implanted defibrillator. Circulation 2004;110:3760–5.

[35] Moss AJ. MADIT II and its implications. Eur Heart J 2003;24(1):16–8.

[36] Le Heuzey J-YF, Chatellier G. 2689 Death causes in a cohort of 2418 patients with an implanted defibrillator: The EVADEF Registry. American Heart Association 2006 Scientific Sessions. Chicago (IL), November 14, 2006.

[37] Stewart GC, Stevenson LW. Patient misperceptions about the survival benefit of implantable defibrillators for primary prevention of death in heart failure. American Heart Association 2006 Scientific Sessions. Chicago (IL), November 12, 2006. Presentation 1877/C135.

[38] Stevenson LW, Desai AS. Selecting patients for discussion of the ICD as primary prevention for sudden death in heart failure. J Card Fail 2006;12:407–12.

ELSEVIER
SAUNDERS

Heart Failure Clin 3 (2007) 245–252

HEART
FAILURE
CLINICS

Burning Questions in Heart Failure Management: Why Do Surgeons and Interventional Cardiologists Talk of Regenerative Cell Therapy?

Warren Sherman, MD, FACC, FSCAI*, Christina Cho, BA,
Timothy P. Martens, MD

College of Physicians & Surgeons, Columbia University, New York, NY, USA

Over the last 20 years, the management of systolic left ventricular dysfunction and congestive heart failure (CHF) has undergone significant changes. Contemporary medical treatment of symptomatic CHF has conferred benefits in functional status and survival [1]. Notably, in the acute setting, percutaneous coronary intervention for ST-elevation myocardial infarction (STEMI) has led to significant reductions in mortality and infarct size [2]. The benefits of percutaneous coronary intervention are also recognized in a subset of patients who had ischemic mitral regurgitation and, more recently, in patients who had post-STEMI shock [3].

Nevertheless, percutaneous coronary intervention has played a minor role in the management of chronic CHF, directed predominantly in patients who have chronic ischemia in regions of viable, yet dysfunctional, myocardium. Advanced devices for intraprocedure hemodynamic support have further enabled interventionalists to perform high-risk percutaneous coronary intervention in patients who have CHF or who are at risk for developing such with even minimal degrees of transient ischemia. Interventionalists based at the cardiac transplant centers are more likely to treat such patients, as well as those who have transplant vasculopathy. Cardiac surgeons are more often confronted with CHF, secondary to valvular heart disease, and their management skills are

accordingly reflected, especially in the perioperative setting. Such is also the case for left ventricular reconstruction procedures (Dor, and others). These clinical demographics are reflected in fellowship training programs for interventional cardiology and cardiothoracic surgery, which do not incorporate dedicated CHF training into core requirements. Clinical competencies for certification by the American Board of Internal Medicine in Interventional Cardiology [4] (minimum of 250 therapeutic interventional cardiac procedures during 12 months) and American Board of Thoracic Surgery [5] (75 cases in adult cardiac are now required: 20 acquired valvular, 40 myocardial revascularization, 20 others, including reoperations) are in keeping with this. For all these reasons, in the day-to-day practice of the interventionalist, CHF is infrequently managed and rarely an indication for percutaneous intervention.

The authors' understanding of myocardial repair is that the heart lacks significant endogenous regenerative potential. This is arguable; to ensure a lifetime of durable myocardial function, cell turnover and repair mechanisms understood to occur in other organ systems is a logical requirement for the heart as well. This would mean that every cell type found within the myocardium, including vascular, muscular, and interstitial, undergoes either replication or replacement throughout postnatal growth and development. The longstanding paradigm of quiescence in postinjury myocardium has been challenged by increased cell-cycle activity observed in the peri-infarction borderzone early after STEMI [6]. Moreover, cardiac stem cells have been isolated from adult hearts

* Corresponding author. Center for Interventional Therapies, Columbia University Medical Center, New York, NY 10032.

E-mail address: ws2157@columbia.edu (W. Sherman).

[7], and cells from remote locations also integrate into vascular and muscular tissue.

Nevertheless, the adult heart has shown a remarkable incapacity for self-repair following myocardial injury. The nature and degree of myocardial injury may influence the potential for regeneration. Acute ischemic injury elicits an early (within hours of coronary occlusion) cascade of events. Within the ischemic zone, cell lysis leads to the release of potent mediators of inflammation and cell migration. Cells not experiencing early death are subject to apoptosis during subsequent weeks. The early re-establishment of coronary flow mitigates and accelerates these processes. During the following 2 weeks, granulation tissue develops, later to be replaced by fibrosis. In areas adjacent to the infarction, cardiomyocytes enter the cell cycle with a frequency greater than observed either within the infarct zone or in areas more remote. Residual normal myocardium demonstrates reactive hyperkinesis immediately following injury, followed closely by progressive myocyte hypertrophy. With time, areas of previously normal myocardium may experience apoptotic myocyte death and fibrosis, resulting in a disadvantageous dilatation, or "remodeling," closely mimicking a pattern seen in states of chronic hemodynamic overload [8]. In postinfarction myocardium, remodeling is susceptible to the effects of inadequate vascular supply, and the role of extracellular matrix in regulating remodeling has also been demonstrated [9]. Irrespective of the mechanism of myocyte depletion, ventricular fibrosis ensues, characterized by a compact meshwork of fibrocytes and extracellular matrix. Tissue density is high and capillary density is low, although typically the postinfarction scar is variably heterogeneous, often containing scattered islands of viable cardiomyocytes. Various aspects of these "irrevocable" processes may be vulnerable to modification, the potential for which has been noted by clinical investigators in surgical and interventional communities. Thus, treatment choices of CHF due to left ventricular dysfunction may not be limited to those that optimize loading conditions and reduce arrhythmia risk.

Brief overview of specific cell types for myocardial repair

A wide range of cell types has been investigated in preclinical studies to identify those for potential use in humans: embryonic stem cells [10,11], fetal [12] and adult [13] cardiomyocytes, smooth muscle cells [14], immortalized myoblasts [15], and adult stem cells. Much research in cell replacement has focused on this last group of cells. As the term is presently used, adult stem cells are cells isolated from various adult tissues that demonstrate the capacity to transform into other cell types or tissue. Specifically included in the category of adult stem cells (ASCs) are skeletal myoblasts [16], bone marrow–derived cells (mesenchymal [17], mononuclear [18], and hematopoetic), circulating progenitor cells [19], and adipose cells [20]. ASCs are further identified and categorized by their expression of surface cellular differentiation (CD) proteins. The presence of CD34 and CD45 identifies a population capable of hematopoiesis and angiogenesis [18,19], whereas CD133 and CD117 (c-kit) are identifiers of multipotent stem cells. Cells expressing these markers can be found in adipose [20] and other tissues.

Preclinical studies

The basic studies relating to all cell lines previously listed are not reviewed herein. Rather, cell types that have entered or are soon to enter clinical trials are highlighted. Ischemic myocardial injury secondary to acute coronary occlusion, either with or without reperfusion, has been the predominant model employed in preclinical cell-therapy studies. This model enables the evaluation of cell replacement at all stages of postinfarction ventricular recovery. Excluded from this approach are such clinical conditions as chronic ischemia without infarction ("hibernating" ventricular dysfunction) and nonischemic myocardial disease, from which limited data are presently available.

The maximal benefit of cell administration would be expected to arise from those precursors capable of generating all three tissues. Thus far, it has been a tall order for any single or multiple cell preparation to achieve true cardiomyogenesis. Therefore, cells destined to become cardiomyocytes would be expected to impart the greatest effect. Nonetheless, improvement in ventricular function has been observed with several different cell types, even those with no demonstrable capacity for cardiomyogenic differentiation.

Skeletal myoblasts

Skeletal myoblasts (SM) have experienced the broadest preclincal and clinical study. Located at the periphery of skeletal muscle bundles, they are cells that serve to replenish skeletal myocytes lost to injury or other causes of cell turnover. They are autologous, mature, and easy to procure. They are identifiable by their expression of desmin and CD56. Procurement of autologous SM entails a three-staged process: (1) open skeletal muscle biopsy, often from the vastus lateralis; (2) physical separation of autologous SM by tissue mincing, decollagenation, and centrifugation; and (3) culture in serum-based media. To attain 10^7 to 10^8 cells, numbers commonly used in implantation studies, 2 to 3 weeks of culturing is required. Once harvested, an aliquot of cells can be evaluated for "potency" by observing their capacity to develop myotubes in vitro, a feature that may predict in vivo efficacy. In animal studies, autologous SM [21] exhibit limited survival following direct implantation into either normal or diseased tissue, with fewer than 20% of cells surviving beyond 24 hours [22]. Surviving autologous SM are capable of further division, maturation, fusion, and engraftment, properties that have been demonstrated in animals [23] and humans [24]. In animal studies, the resultant grafts resemble a histochemical hybrid of skeletal and cardiac muscle, displaying beta myosin heavy chain and developing slow-twitch characteristics [23]. A fatigue-resistant augmentation of diastolic and systolic function has been demonstrated following implantation into areas of chronic infarction [25,26].

Bone marrow–derived cells

Several adult stem cells reside within the bone marrow, contained primarily within the mononuclear population. Included here are the so-called "mesenchymal cells," as well as those identified only by their CD markers. As used investigatively, bone marrow–derived cells have been either autologous or allogeneic, are of varying maturity, and are easily procured. Isolation entails a two- or three-staged process, the first of which involves a standard bone marrow aspiration (50–100 mL from a single puncture). Monnuclear cells can then be isolated by a density gradient technique [27], leading to a mixed population of CD34+, CD45+, and CD133+ cells, along with an assortment of others. Alternatively, bone marrow can be processed in a way so as to select for cells with specific surface markers. In one such technique, bone marrow cells are incubated with ferromagnetic particles to which monoclonal antibodies have been conjugated. Antibodies to specific markers, such as CD133, can be used to target cells expressing that particular antigen. Bound cells are then separated magnetically. By either this or the density gradient technique, yields of between 10^6 and 10^8 cells are common.

Within the bone marrow mononuclear population are cells referred to as "mesenchymal" [17]. They are isolatable by virtue of their physical adherence to plastic and their ability to follow several different maturation pathways [17]. They do not uniformly express specific surface markers, although they are reported to be positive for CD105, CD166, CD29, and CD44 and negative for CD34 and CD45. Human mesenchymal cells were reported to differentiate into cardiomyocytes after implantation into murine hearts [28] and to integrate into muscular and vascular tissues of infracted rat myocardium [29]. Several types of mesenchymal lineage cells have been described (mesenchymal stem cells, mesenchymal progenitor cells, multi-potent adult progenitor cells) and tested in preclinical models. Given that they often have overlapping expression profiles of various cell surface markers, the distinction between types is sometimes unclear.

The true cardiogenic potential of bone marrow–derived cells is controversial. Early data [30] suggesting the integration of these cells into infracted murine myocardium has been questioned [31,32]. At issue is whether the present observations are explained by any one or more of two processes: transdifferentiation to new cardiomyocytes or fusion with resident cardiomyocytes [33,34], or impart benefit to the injured heart by other mechanisms. The functional consequence of bone marrow cell integration is subject to ongoing study.

Cell-delivery techniques

There are three methods for the delivery of cells to the left ventricle: (1) direct implantation, (2) local vascular infusion, and (3) induced systemic release. Surgical techniques, developed during proof-of-concept studies and adapted for clinical studies, are all performed through the epicardial surface either alone or in combination with adjunctive coronary artery bypass graft, LVAD implantation, or other procedures. On the other hand, catheter-injection techniques have largely been performed as sole interventions [35].

Direct implantation techniques involve the intramural placement of cells under direct visualization of the surgically exposed heart or with intravascular catheter delivery systems. Catheter-injection systems for direct implantation are "specialized" devices that permit either endocardial or transepicardial injection. Other catheters systems, some of which use the coronary venous system [36], are also under investigation for extravascular administration.

Intracoronary infusion makes use of coronary arterial procedures already integrated into clinical practice. The patency and flow characteristics of the target coronary bed and the propensity of the cell preparation to adhere and transmigrate to the target tissue places specific requirements onto this method. The interrelationships between cell and vessel wall, and operative signaling mechanisms between target tissue and injected cells bear heavily on tissue levels. Although intracoronary administration typically uses standard "over-the-wire" balloon angioplasty catheters and is easy to employ, problems with cell retention [37] and intravascular aggregation and thrombosis [38] have been reported.

Lastly, there is evidence that cells from remote anatomic locations are capable of being incorporated into the myocardium. In animals given granulocyte colony stimulating factor and stem cell factor, bone marrow–derived cells were found in myocytes, endothelial cells, and smooth muscle cells within arteriole walls, at the perimeter of the infarction [39]. Following experimental infarction, endothelial progenitor cells mobilized with granulocyte colony stimulating factor are capable of limiting ventricular remodeling and apoptosis through neovascularization [18]. Bone marrow–derived cells have been identified in postmortem hearts following sex-mismatched bone marrow transplantation [40].

Clinical studies that influence current thinking

In assessing the therapeutic potential of stem cells, it is important to emphasize the pitfalls of the current methodologies. First, few methods of cell processing or delivery are standardized. The interstudy variability of each is substantial. Second, a high rate of early cell attrition is unavoidable, irrespective of cell characteristics or delivery method. Consequently, dose ranges for efficacy and toxicity have not been established, and it stands to reason that both may be significantly affected by improvements in cell retention.

The number of clinical studies in cell therapy for cardiovascular disease is steadily increasing, and the field has entered the era of controlled trials. Three clinical subsets have been targeted: those who have STEMI, those who have CHF, and those who have CMI. Herein, the authors address two of them: STEMI and CHF due to systolic left ventricular dysfunction.

Acute myocardial infarction

The management of patients who have acute myocardial infarction (MI) by medical stabilization and early revascularization may have a potential adjunct in the early administration of cell injections. In three studies [41–43], subjects who had STEMI treated with acute coronary stenting were given either bone marrow–derived or peripheral-derived mononuclear cells. Cells were administered 4 to 10 days postinfarction, a delay that enabled early clinical stabilization and sufficient time for cell procurement, through an over-the-wire balloon catheter during intermittent coronary occlusion. From these studies, feasibility, safety, and preliminary efficacy (increments in ejection fraction of 4–7% at 4–6 months) were established. Effects of ventricular remodeling and infarct size were also suggested by these and other [44] studies.

Alternative strategies for recruiting regenerative cells into the zone of acute myocardial infarction are also under clinical investigation, including the administration of granulocyte colony stimulating factor for bone marrow cell mobilization.

Chronic myocardial disease

Cell therapy for chronic myocardial disease entered clinical study 7 years ago when a patient who had CHF and coronary disease underwent direct transepicardial autologous skeletal myoblasts (ASM) implantation at the time of coronary artery bypass surgery [45]. Since that time, over 300 adjunct-to-cardiac surgery cell implantation procedures have been performed worldwide [24,46–48]. All reported studies have sought to demonstrate feasibility and safety. Most of the subjects enrolled have had chronic stable CHF (New York Heart Association [NYHA] class 2–4) and poor left ventricular function (ejection fraction [EF] between 15%–40%) due to ischemic myocardial disease [24,46–50]. One study [48] enrolled patients who had more recent MI (10 days to 3 months) and no CHF or poor ventricular function (EF between 40%–60%). All studies employed direct transepicardial implantation techniques at the time of either bypass surgery [24,46,47] or left ventricular assist device implantation [24]. Cell type (autologous skeletal myoblasts versus bone marrow–derived CD133+ cells versus CD34+ cells) and number (10 million–1.2 billion), region of implantation (infarct versus peri-infarct), and revascularization protocol (coronary bypass grafting to cell implantation zone versus none) were different. Proof of myocardial nonviability was a requirement in only one study [46]. Although early postprocedure safety data were marked by increased incidence of ventricular arrhythmias [46], such has not been a widespread observation. Preventative measures have been adopted by some [47,51], and most recent data seriously question the existence of any relationship between ventricular arrhythmias and ASM implantation [49].

Efficacy data from early trials supported benefits in both symptoms (a 1–2 grade drop in NYHA class) and ventricular function (increments in regional and global ventricular function of between 10%–30% [47]. The mechanism of improvement has not been elucidated; improvements in systolic ventricular function in the regions of autologous SM implantation were described [46]. A multicenter study, the Myoblast Autologous Grafting in Ischemic Cardiomayopathy (MAGIC) Trial [49], represented the first randomized placebo-controlled assessment of the efficacy of surgical skeletal myoblast implantation for patients who had severe heart failure. Eligibility criteria were patients who presented with NYHA heart-failure class II or III and EF 35% or less, and a prior MI with residual akinetic and nonviable scar, and were indicated for concomitant coronary artery bypass graft in remote viable but ischemic myocardium. Between 2002 and 2006, 120 patients were enrolled, with 97 receiving one of two doses (400×10^6 or 800×10^6) of cultured autologous skeletal myoblasts, and the remaining subjects constituting the placebo arm. All subjects were implanted with automatic implantable cardioverter defibrillator and underwent Holter monitoring to evaluate arrhythmia risk, and preliminary safety data indicated that SM transplantation gave rise to no additional arrhythmic risk. The final results, reported November 2006 [49], showed no difference in the primary efficacy end-point (regional echocardiographic wall motion score) but significant improvements in radionuclide EF in the high-dose treatment group. The subjects in the high-dose group also exhibited an end-systolic volume decrease 15% greater than that recorded among the placebo subjects.

Studies have been conducted with catheter-based delivery for chronic myocardial disease [52–55]. The clinical populations are similar to those of the surgical studies (NYHA class 2–4 CHF due to ischemic systolic left ventricular dysfunction) but are not candidates for mechanical revascularization. Therefore, the only intervention in most of these studies was cell implantation, by either intramyocardial or intracoronary infusion. Depending on the degree of viable versus nonviable myocardium, myogenic (ASM) or angiogenic cell products, respectively, were administered. The results are encouraging in terms of the technical feasibility and safety of this injection strategy, and efficacy with regard to ventricular function is suggestive of improvement (EF increment of 4%–5% along with greater wall thickening in the implanted zones).

The second report [54,55] describes a small series of patients that received direct catheter-based implantation of bone marrow mononuclear cells. Subjects had NYHA class 2–3 CHF, myocardial ischemia on nuclear imaging, reduced left ventricular EF (<40%), and coronary disease unsuitable for revascularization. A mixed population of bone marrow mononuclear cells (30×10^6, CD45+ and CD34+) were injected into the ischemic areas. There were no safety or logistic problems, and improvement in ventricular ischemia and function were observed. Both of these studies are small (a total of 19 patients enrolled).

Physician attitudes to stem cell research and "therapy"

Numerous polls clearly demonstrate the evolution of public opinion of stem cell research toward one of embracing its medical potential. Nearly all such data reflect attitudes toward embryonic stem cell research, with little attention focused on adult-derived progenitor cells, which is of course the category of cells used in essentially all clinical studies of cardiovascular disease to date. Summary reports and opinions as to the clinical benefits of adult stem cells reflect the authors' backgrounds and interpretations of published data [56], not necessarily the thinking of broader constituencies [57]. Polling data of cardiovascular specialists are not to be found. The closest approximation in the United States can be found in a web-based survey of the general physician community [58], taken before a 2006 US Senate vote on a bill to ease restrictions on federal funding of embryonic stem cell research. As was the case in a 2004 poll, the vast majority of physicians favored passage of the bill (HR 801).

Several indirect indicators of opinion within the cardiac surgical and interventional communities are available. The European Society of Cardiology convened a task force to review the status of clinical investigation into cardiac repair with autologous ASCs. Its consensus statement [59], formulated by investigators who are leaders in the field, is a balanced and thoughtful appraisal. Also, over the past 5 years, attendance at clinically oriented meetings on cell-based cardiac repair has been steadily increasing and paralleled the accumulation of clinical trial data.

Summary

That cardiac regeneration is remotely feasible, elicits thoughts of curing one of the most debilitating of human diseases. The term *stem cell* brings to the surface many hopes, and concerns, among physicians and the public alike, both of which have come to expect frequent advances in medical therapeutics. The evolution of public opinion toward embryonic stem cell research is clear and positive, and, unfortunately, overshadows, even confuses, that of adult stem cells, despite their use in essentially all clinical studies of cardiovascular disease to date. Strange, perhaps, that the voices of cardiovascular specialists are not to be heard.

The premise that an influx of new cells will reverse ventricular dysfunction, or prevent its progression, has found solid support in animal studies. From data in hand, one can conclude that the implantation of cells into diseased myocardium can be accomplished safely and without a great deal of technical difficulty. Small-to-modest changes in ventricular function can be expected from cell replacement techniques in patients who have chronic myocardial disease. Clinical correlations of such changes are not established at this time. The field is now entering a phase of design and execution of efficacy trials to test clinical outcomes, as well as to substantiate observed changes in left ventricular function. As much as is practical, trials need to be designed to evaluate cell replacement as the sole intervention, rather than in combination with other therapies. The choice of cell type, dose, and delivery technique, and matching these with underlying myocardial disease will be key in the formulation of treatment arms. For patients who have CHF, objective measures of symptom improvement and parameters of quality of life are incorporated into trial designs. Changes in ejection fraction must be correlated to other parameters of ventricular function, such as regional wall thickening and motion, that may better reflect the biologic effects of cells.

The authors suspect that cell implantation will find a role in clinical practice. In patients who have STEMI, implantation of cells that facilitate angiogenesis may preserve surviving cardiomyocytes and retard ventricular remodeling. However, limiting cardiomyocyte loss through angiogenesis will fall short of the goal of cardiomyocyte replacement. For this, the implantation of myogenic cells will be necessary, though coadministration with vasculogenic cells may increase perfusion and therefore survival of myogenic. For patients who have chronic myocardial disease, the challenges are greater. The tissue environment is unwelcoming to implanted cells, and new approaches to facilitating cell survival are in the making. So, absent competed pivotal trials, the muted public reaction of interventional cardiologists and cardiac surgeons to regenerative cell therapy is understandable. Nevertheless, we talk of regenerative therapy in enthusiastic terms, as cell transfer holds a profound conceptual advantage over existing therapies in its potential for restoring ventricular function. It is now a matter of translation.

References

[1] Jessup M, Brozena S. Heart failure. N Engl J Med 2003;348(20):2007–18.

[2] Fox KAA, Steg PG, Eagle KA, et al. Decline in Rates of Death and Heart Failure in Acute Coronary Syndromes, 1999–2006. JAMA 2007;297(17): 1892–900.

[3] Hochman JS, Sleeper LA, Webb JG, et al. Early revascularization and long-term survival in cardiogenic shock complicating acute myocardial infarction. JAMA 2006;295(21):2511–5.

[4] Medicine ABoI. Policies and Procedures for Certification. Pliladelphia: ABIM; 2006.

[5] Surgery ABoT. Operative Case Requrements. 2002.

[6] Beltrami AP, Urbanek K, Kajstura J, et al. Evidence that human cardiac myocytes divide after myocardial infarction. N Engl J Med 2001;344(23):1750–7.

[7] Smith RR, Barile L, Cho HC, et al. Regenerative potential of cardiosphere-derived cells expanded from percutaneous endomyocardial biopsy specimens. Circulation 2007;115(7):896–908.

[8] Jackson BM, Gorman JH, Moainie SL, et al. Extension of borderzone myocardium in postinfarction dilated cardiomyopathy. J Am Coll Cardiol 2002; 40(6):1160–7 [discussion: 8–71].

[9] Mann DL, Taegtmeyer H. Dynamic regulation of the extracellular matrix after mechanical unloading of the failing human heart: recovering the missing link in left ventricular remodeling. Circulation 2001;104(10):1089–91.

[10] Maltsev VA, Rohwedel J, Hescheler J, et al. Embryonic stem cells differentiate in vitro into cardiomyocytes representing sinusnodal, atrial and ventricular cell types. Mech Dev 1993;44(1):41–50.

[11] Kehat I, Kenyagin-Karsenti D, Snir M, et al. Human embryonic stem cells can differentiate into myocytes with structural and functional properties of cardiomyocytes. J Clin Invest 2001;108(3):407–14.

[12] Soonpaa MH, Koh GY, Klug MG, et al. Formation of nascent intercalated disks between grafted fetal cardiomyocytes and host myocardium. Science 1994;264(5155):98–101.

[13] Sakai T, Li RK, Weisel RD, et al. Autologous heart cell transplantation improves cardiac function after myocardial injury. Ann Thorac Surg 1999;68(6): 2074–80 [discussion: 80–1].

[14] Li RK, Jia ZQ, Weisel RD, et al. Smooth muscle cell transplantation into myocardial scar tissue improves heart function. J Mol Cell Cardiol 1999;31(3): 513–22.

[15] Koh GY, Klug MG, Soonpaa MH, et al. Differentiation and long-term survival of C2C12 myoblast grafts in heart. J Clin Invest 1993;92(3):1548–54.

[16] Chiu RC, Zibaitis A, Kao RL. Cellular cardiomyoplasty: myocardial regeneration with satellite cell implantation. Ann Thorac Surg 1995;60(1):12–8.

[17] Pittenger MF, Mackay AM, Beck SC, et al. Multilineage potential of adult human mesenchymal stem cells. Science 1999;284(5411):143–7.

[18] Kocher AA, Schuster MD, Szabolcs MJ, et al. Neovascularization of ischemic myocardium by human bone-marrow-derived angioblasts prevents cardiomyocyte apoptosis, reduces remodeling and improves cardiac function. Nat Med 2001;7(4): 430–6.

[19] Kawamoto A, Gwon HC, Iwaguro H, et al. Therapeutic potential of ex vivo expanded endothelial progenitor cells for myocardial ischemia. Circulation 2001;103(5):634–7.

[20] Zuk PA, Zhu M, Mizuno H, et al. Multilineage cells from human adipose tissue: implications for cell-based therapies. Tissue Eng 2001;7(2):211–28.

[21] Qu Z, Balkir L, van Deutekom JCT, et al. Development of approaches to improve cell survival in myoblast transfer therapy. J Cell Biol 1998;142(5): 1257–67.

[22] Muller-Ehmsen J, Whittaker P, Kloner RA, et al. Survival and development of neonatal rat cardiomyocytes transplanted into adult myocardium. J Mol Cell Cardiol 2002;34(2):107–16.

[23] Reinecke H, Zhang M, Bartosek T, et al. Survival, integration, and differentiation of cardiomyocyte grafts: a study in normal and injured rat hearts. Circulation 1999;100(2):193–202.

[24] Pagani FD, DerSimonian H, Zawadzka A, et al. Autologous skeletal myoblasts transplanted to ischemia-damaged myocardium in humans. Histological analysis of cell survival and differentiation. J Am Coll Cardiol 2003;41(5):879–88.

[25] Taylor DA, Atkins BZ, Hungspreugs P, et al. Regenerating functional myocardium: improved performance after skeletal myoblast transplantation. Nat Med 1998;4(8):929–33.

[26] He KL, Yi GH, Sherman W, et al. Autologous skeletal myoblast transplantation improved hemodynamics and left ventricular function in chronic heart failure dogs. J Heart Lung Transplant 2005; 24(11):1940–9.

[27] Boyum A. Isolation of mononuclear cells and granulocytes from human blood. Isolation of monuclear cells by one centrifugation, and of granulocytes by combining centrifugation and sedimentation at 1 g. Scand J Clin Lab Invest Suppl 1968;97:77–89.

[28] Toma C, Pittenger MF, Cahill KS, et al. Human mesenchymal stem cells differentiate to a cardiomyocyte phenotype in the adult murine heart. Circulation 2002;105(1):93–8.

[29] Tomita S, Li RK, Weisel RD, et al. Autologous transplantation of bone marrow cells improves damaged heart function. Circulation 1999;100(Suppl 19): II247–56.

[30] Orlic D, Kajstura J, Chimenti S, et al. Bone marrow cells regenerate infarcted myocardium. Nature 2001; 410(6829):701–5.

[31] Murry CE, Soonpaa MH, Reinecke H, et al. Haematopoietic stem cells do not transdifferentiate into cardiac myocytes in myocardial infarcts. Nature 2004; 428(6983):664–8.

[32] Balsam LB, Wagers AJ, Christensen JL, et al. Haematopoietic stem cells adopt mature haematopoietic fates in ischaemic myocardium. Nature 2004; 428(6983):668–73.

[33] Reinecke H, Minami E, Poppa V, et al. Evidence for fusion between cardiac and skeletal muscle cells. Circ Res 2004;94(6):e56–60.

[34] Nygren JM, Jovinge S, Breitbach M, et al. Bone marrow-derived hematopoietic cells generate cardiomyocytes at a low frequency through cell fusion, but not transdifferentiation. Nat Med 2004;10(5): 494–501.

[35] Sherman W, Martens TP, Viles-Gonzalez JF, et al. Catheter-based delivery of cells to the heart. Nat Clin Pract Cardiovasc Med 2006;1(Suppl 3):S57–64.

[36] Thompson CA, Nasseri BA, Makower J, et al. Percutaneous transvenous cellular cardiomyoplasty. A novel nonsurgical approach for myocardial cell transplantation. J Am Coll Cardiol 2003;41(11): 1964–71.

[37] Hou D, Youssef EA-S, Brinton TJ, et al. Radiolabeled cell distribution after intramyocardial, intracoronary, and interstitial retrograde coronary venous delivery: implications for current clinical trials. Circulation 2005;112(9_Suppl):I-150–6.

[38] Vulliet PR, Greeley M, Halloran SM, et al. Intra-coronary arterial injection of mesenchymal stromal cells and microinfarction in dogs. Lancet 2004; 363(9411):783–4.

[39] Orlic D, Kajstura J, Chimenti S, et al. Mobilized bone marrow cells repair the infarcted heart, improving function and survival. Proc Natl Acad Sci USA 2001;98(18):10344–9.

[40] Deb A, Wang S, Skelding KA, et al. Bone marrow-derived cardiomyocytes are present in adult human heart: a study of gender-mismatched bone marrow transplantation patients. Circulation 2003;107(9): 1247–9.

[41] Assmus B, Schachinger V, Teupe C, et al. Transplantation of progenitor cells and regeneration enhancement in acute myocardial infarction (TOPCARE-AMI). Circulation 2002;106(24):3009–17.

[42] Strauer BE, Brehm M, Zeus T, et al. Repair of infarcted myocardium by autologous intracoronary mononuclear bone marrow cell transplantation in humans. Circulation 2002;106(15):1913–8.

[43] Wollert KC, Meyer GP, Lotz J, et al. Intracoronary autologous bone-marrow cell transfer after myocardial infarction: the BOOST randomised controlled clinical trial. Lancet 2004;364(9429): 141–8.

[44] Janssens S, Dubois C, Bogaert J, et al. Autologous bone marrow-derived stem-cell transfer in patients with ST-segment elevation myocardial infarction: double-blind, randomized controlled trial. Lancet 2006;367(9505):113–21.

[45] Menasche P, Hagege AA, Scorsin M, et al. Myoblast transplantation for heart failure. Lancet 2001; 357(9252):279–80.

[46] Menasche P, Hagege AA, Vilquin JT, et al. Autologous skeletal myoblast transplantation for severe postinfarction left ventricular dysfunction. J Am Coll Cardiol 2003;41(7):1078–83.

[47] Herreros J, Prosper F, Perez A, et al. Autologous intramyocardial injection of cultured skeletal muscle-derived stem cells in patients with non-acute myocardial infarction. Eur Heart J 2003;24(22): 2012–20.

[48] Stamm C, Westphal B, Kleine HD, et al. Autologous bone-marrow stem-cell transplantation for myocardial regeneration. Lancet 2003;361(9351):45–6.

[49] Menasche P. The MAGIC trial. American Heart Association scientific sessions. Chicago: 2006; in press.

[50] Patel AN, Geffner L, Vina RF, et al. Surgical treatment for congestive heart failure with autologous adult stem cell transplantation: a prospective randomized study. J Thorac Cardiovasc Surg 2005; 130(6):1631–8.

[51] Dib N, Michler RE, Pagani FD, et al. Safety and feasibility of autologous myoblast transplantation in patients with ischemic cardiomyopathy: four-year follow-up. Circulation 2005;112(12):1748–55.

[52] Sherman W, Chronos N, Ellis S, et al. Intramyocardial myoblast treatment for ischemic heart failure: results of a phase 1 study. J Card Fail 2006;12(6 Suppl 1):S74.

[53] Siminiak T, Fiszer D, Jerzykowska O, et al. Percutaneous autologous myoblast transplantation in the treatment of post-infarction myocardial contractility impairment–report on two cases. Kardiol Pol 2003;59(12):492–501.

[54] Perin EC, Dohmann HF, Borojevic R, et al. Transendocardial, autologous bone marrow cell transplantation for severe, chronic ischemic heart failure. Circulation 2003;107(18):2294–302.

[55] Smits PC, van Geuns RJ, Poldermans D, et al. Catheter-based intramyocardial injection of autologous skeletal myoblasts as a primary treatment of ischemic heart failure: clinical experience with six-month follow-up. J Am Coll Cardiol 2003;42(12):2063–9.

[56] Prentice D. Adult stem cells, appendix K in monitoring stem cell research: a report of the president's council on bioethics. Washington, DC: Government Printing Office; 2004. p. 309–46.

[57] Smith S, Neaves W, Teitelbaum S. Adult stem cell treatments for diseases? Science 2006;313(5786):439.

[58] Physicians Strongly In Favor of Embryonic Stem Cell Research; Overwhelming Majority Support Increased Federal Funding. In: Stem Cell Newscom; 2006. Available at: http://www.stemcellnews.com/articles/physicians-support-embryonic-stem-cell-research.htm.

[59] Bartunek J, Dimmeler S, Drexler H, et al. The consensus of the task force of the European Society of Cardiology concerning the clinical investigation of the use of autologous adult stem cells for repair of the heart. Eur Heart J 2006;27(11):1338–40.

**ELSEVIER
SAUNDERS**

Heart Failure Clin 3 (2007) 253–257

**HEART
FAILURE
CLINICS**

Index

Note: Page numbers of article titles are in **boldface** type.

Moving?

Make sure your subscription moves with you!

To notify us of your new address, find your **Clinics Account Number** (located on your mailing label above your name), and contact customer service at:

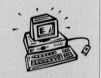

E-mail: elspcs@elsevier.com

800-654-2452 (subscribers in the U.S. & Canada)
407-345-4000 (subscribers outside of the U.S. & Canada)

Fax number: 407-363-9661

Elsevier Periodicals Customer Service
6277 Sea Harbor Drive
Orlando, FL 32887-4800

*To ensure uninterrupted delivery of your subscription, please notify us at least 4 weeks in advance of move.

ELSEVIER